RECENT ADVANCES IN

Paediatrics

Blackwells.
39109
£23-36

D0496317

RECENT ADVANCES IN PAEDIATRICS

Contents of Number 11
Edited by T.J. David

ISBN 0443 047537

You can place your order by contacting your local medical bookseller or the Sales Promotion Department, Robert Stevenson House, 1–3 Baxter's Place, Leith Walk, Edinburgh EH1 3AF, UK

Tel: (031) 556 2424; Telex: 727511 LONGMN G; Fax (031) 558 1278

Look out for *Recent Advances in Paediatrics 13* in November 1994

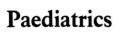

Paediatrics

Edited by

T. J. David MD PhD FRCP DCH

Professor, and Head,
Department of Child Health,
University of Manchester;
Honorary Consultant Paediatrician,
Booth Hall Children's Hospital,
Manchester, UK

NUMBER TWELVE

CHURCHILL LIVINGSTONE
EDINBURGH LONDON MADRID MELBOURNE MILAN NEW YORK AND TOKYO 1994

CHURCHILL LIVINGSTONE
Medical Division of Longman Group UK Limited

Distributed in the United States of America by
Churchill Livingstone Inc., 650 Avenue of the Americas,
New York, N.Y. 10011, and by associated companies,
branches and representatives throughout the world.

First published 1994

ISBN 0-443-048711

ISSN 0-309-0140

British Library Cataloguing in Publication Data
A CIP catalogue record for this book is available from the
British Library

Library of Congress Cataloguing in Publication Data is
available

The
publisher's
policy is to use
paper manufactured
from sustainable forests

Produced by Longman Singapore Pte Ltd
Printed in Singapore

Contents

Preface

The aim of *Recent Advances in Paediatrics* is to provide a review of important topics and help doctors keep abreast of developments in the subject. The book is intended for the practising clinican and the postgraduate student. There are 13 chapters on a variety of general paediatric and neonatal topics. The selection of topics has veered towards those of general rather than special interest.

The final chapter, an annotated literature review, is a personal selection of key articles and useful reviews published in 1992. As with the choice of subjects for the main chapters, the selection of articles has inclined towards those of general rather than special interest. There is, however, special emphasis on community paediatrics and tropical paediatrics, as these two important areas are sometimes poorly covered in general paediatric journals. Trying to reduce to an acceptable size the short-list of particularly interesting articles is an especially difficult task. To assist I try to avoid unnecessary duplication of a topic, so, for example, there are no major sections on HIV infection or malaria in this year's literature review, as these are covered separately in two chapters. Each year brings its own curious small rush of papers in particular topics; this year there has been unusual interest in bicycle helmets, retinopathy of prematurity, antibiotic-resistant pneumococci, and the adverse effects of exposure to lead.

Annual publication of this series provides the opportunity to respond to the wishes of readers, and any suggestions for topics to be included in future issues are always welcome. Please write to me at the address below.

I am indebted to the authors for their hard work, prompt delivery of manuscripts and patience in dealing with my queries and requests. I would also like to thank Yvonne O'Leary of Churchill Livingstone for all her help, my personal assistant Valerie Smith for her help with the literature database, and my wife and sons for all their support.

Professor T. J. David   1994
University Department of Child Health
Booth Hall Children's Hospital
Manchester M9 2AA
UK

Contributors

Frank N. Bamford MD DCH DPH FFPHM FRCP
Reader in Developmental Paediatrics, Manchester University,
Manchester, UK

P. G. Chait MB BCh FF RAD(D)SA FRCR(C) FRCP(C) DABR
Assistant Professor, Department of Diagnostic Imaging,
University of Toronto; Staff Radiologist, Hospital for Sick Children,
Toronto, Ontario, Canada

Howard M. Corneli MD
Associate Professor of Pediatrics, University of Utah College of Medicine;
Co-Director, Emergency Services, Primary Children's Medical Center,
Salt Lake City, Utah, USA

Jonathan M. Couriel MA MB BChir FRCP
Consultant in Paediatrics and Paediatric Respiratory Medicine,
Booth Hall Children's Hospital, Manchester, UK

T. J. David MD PhD FRCP DCH
Professor, and Head, Department of Child Health, University of
Manchester; Honorary Consultant Paediatrician, Booth Hall Children's
Hospital, Manchester, UK

Kay E. Davies MA DPhil
Professor, Molecular Genetics Group, Institute of Molecular Medicine,
John Radcliffe Hospital, Oxford, UK

Karen Dunnell BSc MA (Hon)MFPHM
Head of Health Statistics, Office of Population Censuses and Surveys,
London, UK

Diana Gibb MB ChB MRCP(Paed) MD MSc(Epidem)
Senior Lecturer in Epidemiology, and Honorary Consultant Paediatrician,
Epidemiology and Biostatistics Unit, Institute of Child Health,
London, UK

Brian Greenwood MD FRCP
Director, MRC Laboratories, Fajara, Banjul, The Gambia, Africa

John E. Grunow MD
Associate Professor of Pediatrics, University of Oklahoma Health Sciences
Center, Oklahoma City, Oklahoma, USA

Mark C. Hirst BSc PhD
Senior Research Fellow, Molecular Genetics Group, Institute of Molecular
Medicine, John Radcliffe Hospital, Oxford, UK

Sheila M. Innis PhD
Associate Professor, Department of Paediatrics, University of British
Columbia, Vancouver, Canada

George H. McCracken Jr AB MD
Professor of Pediatrics, The Sarah M. and Charles E. Seay Chair in
Pediatric Infectious Diseases, University of Texas Southwestern Medical
Center, Dallas, Texas, USA

Carrie Mullan MSc RPDt
Clinical Dietitian, Hospital for Sick Children, Toronto, Ontario, Canada

Marie-Louise Newell MB MSc PhD
Coordinator, European Collaborative Study, Department of Paediatric
Epidemiology, Institute of Child Health, London, UK

Paul B. Pencharz MB ChB PhD FRCP(C)
Professor of Paediatrics and Nutrition, University of Toronto; Head,
Division of Clinical Nutrition, Hospital for Sick Children, Toronto,
Ontario, Canada

Lewis Rosenbloom MB FRCP DCH
Consultant Paediatric Neurologist, Royal Liverpool Children's NHS Trust,
Alder Hey Hospital, Liverpool, UK

Xavier Sáez-Llorens MD
Professor of Pediatrics and Infectious Diseases, University of Panama,
School of Medicine, Hospital del Niño of Panama, Republic of Panama

Sue Savoie RN
Nutrition Support Nurse, Gastrostomy Clinic, Hospital for Sick Children,
Toronto, Ontario, Canada

Graham R. Serjeant MD FRCP
Director, MRC Laboratories, University of the West Indies, Kingston,
Jamaica, West Indies

Mortality, morbidity and health-related behaviour in childhood

K. Dunnell

In 1989 the Department of Health set up a Central Health Monitoring Unit (CHMU) to draw together the wide variety of information available about health. It is a central information source for policy makers. As an important provider of information the Office of Population Censuses and Surveys (OPCS) works closely with the CHMU. One collaborative project was an epidemiological review of child health. This included producing a guide to centrally available statistics relating to the health of children, which was published with a summary article.[1] This chapter updates and extends that article. It illustrates the way the statistics can be used by presenting a selection of OPCS data covering three aspects of health — mortality, morbidity and health-related behaviour. Infant (under 1 year) mortality and morbidity are not covered specifically.

MORTALITY

Table 1.1 gives the 1991 all-cause death rates for males and females in different age groups. It shows the comparatively high risk of death in infancy

Table1.1   Age-specific death rates for males and females — 1991 as a percentage of the 1981 rate (rates per 1000 population, births for those under the age of 1)

Age (years)	Males		Females	
	1991 rate	% of 1981	1991 rate	% of 1981
Under 1	8.30	66	6.40	68
1–4	0.40	75	0.33	72
5–9	0.21	78	0.16	84
10–14	0.23	79	0.15	79
15–19	0.69	84	0.28	88
20–24	0.86	104	0.33	94
25–34	0.94	106	0.45	87
35–44	1.76	96	1.06	84
45–54	4.62	76	2.91	77
55–64	13.80	78	8.10	85
65–74	38.50	84	22.00	91
75–84	93.60	89	58.60	89
85 +	197.10	87	163.80	90

and the very low risk between the ages of 5 and 14. Thereafter, risk of death rises for each subsequent age group. The table also shows that in the first year of life boys have a death rate significantly higher than that of girls. This difference between the sexes continues throughout life. Thus in 1990 males had a life expectancy at birth of 73 years, females one of 78 years.

The table also shows for each age and sex group the proportional value of the 1991 rate compared with the 1981 rate. It can be seen that infants and children have generally experienced greater improvements in mortality than older age groups. Infant mortality has improved the most, with rates for both boys and girls being only two-thirds of their 1981 value. The rates for boys and girls aged 10–14 were four-fifths of their 1981 value — a greater improvement than for almost all the older age groups. In general, mortality improved by a similar amount for both boys and girls.

There has been little change in the main causes of death in the last 20 years. The percentage distribution of the main causes is shown in the columns on deaths in Table 1.2. Death from injury and poisoning is the commonest cause of death in children aged 5–14 — more than one-third of deaths in this age group. Cancer is the cause of almost one-quarter of deaths among children aged 5–14; diseases of the nervous system and sense organs are responsible for 1 in 10.

Among younger children aged between 28 days and 4 years one-third of deaths fall into the category of signs, symptoms and ill-defined conditions — mostly deaths from sudden infant death syndrome arising in the postneonatal period. Congenital malformations account for almost 1 in 5 deaths under the age of 5.

From Table 1.1 we have seen that at all ages, including infancy, males have higher death rates than females. This applies to most of the major causes of death but most particularly to deaths from injury and poisoning. This is reflected in the percentage distribution of causes of death in Table 1.2. Injury and poisoning caused 41% of deaths of boys aged 5–14, but only 30% of deaths of girls in the same age group.

Although injury and poisoning are the major cause of death for children aged 1 year or more, there have been considerable improvements over the last 20 years. Mortality rates for both boys and girls aged 1–4 and 5–9 have generally halved. Those for older children have shown smaller improvements. Death rates from cancer have also decreased among all age groups of children. Detailed statistics about children's mortality are published each year.[2–4]

MORBIDITY AND DISABILITY

OPCS has carried out the General Household Survey (GHS) continuously since 1971.[5]

The survey asks parents of children about their children's health and provides three measures of morbidity — long-standing illness, limitation of

Table 1.2 Percentage distribution of the main causes of death (1990), hospital admissions (1985) and general practitioners (GP) consultations (1982)

	Deaths (%)		Admissions (%)		Consultations (%)	
	28 days-4 years	5–14 years	0–4 years	5–14 years	0–4 years	5–14 years
All causes						
Boys	100	100	100	100	100	100
Girls	100	100	100	100	100	100
All children	100	100	100	100	100	100
Disease of respiratory system						
Boys	8	5	24	19	31	33
Girls	9	3	20	23	29	31
All children	9	4	22	20	30	32
Disease of digestive system						
Boys	1	1	8	9	3	2
Girls	2	1	7	9	3	2
All children	1	1	8	9	3	2
Nervous system and sense organs						
Boys	8	10	7	12	16	14
Girls	7	11	8	14	15	15
All children	7	11	7	12	16	14
Perinatal						
Boys	7	0	12	0	0	0
Girls	7	1	15	0	0	0
All children	7	0	13	0	0	0
Injury and poisoning						
Boys	11	42	10	22	3	9
Girls	9	30	11	17	3	7
All children	10	37	11	20	3	8
Signs, symptoms and ill-defined conditions						
Boys	33	0	16	13	9	11
Girls	32	0	18	15	10	11
All children	32	0	17	14	9	11
Congenital malformations						
Boys	16	6	7	7	1	0
Girls	19	10	7	4	0	0
All children	17	8	7	6	0	0
Cancer						
Boys	4	21	1	2	0	0
Girls	4	26	1	3	0	0
All children	4	23	1	2	0	0
Other						
Boys	11	14	14	17	37	31
Girls	12	17	13	16	40	35
All children	12	15	14	17	38	33
Totals						
Boys	1971	671	26 382	21 684	52 280	47 880
Girls	1399	450	17 572	14 965	44 538	46 567
All children	3370	1121	43 954	36 649	96 818	94 447

activity arising from long-standing illness and restricted activity arising from illness in the 2 weeks before interview.

Figure 1.1 shows the proportions of children with the different types of reported morbidity from 1981 to 1990.

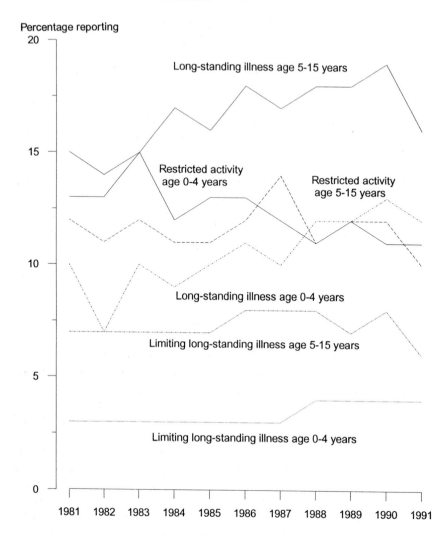

Fig. 1.1   Trends in morbidity shown by age and category, in Great Britain. Data from the General Household Survey, years 1981–1991.[5]

In contrast to mortality trends, there is no evidence that the health of children, as perceived by their parents, improved during the 1980s. There is some suggestion that rates of long-standing illness among children aged 5–15 increased.

In recent years almost 1 in 5 children aged 5–15 were reported as suffering from a long-standing illness, although only about one-half of them had a resulting limitation in activities. The figures for children in 1991 aged 0–4 were 12% with a long-standing illness, and 4% with a limiting long-standing illness. While the rates of long-standing illness appeared to have increased over the last 10 years, illness in the last 2 weeks was reported for about 1 in 10 children in both age groups consistently during the 1980s.

In 1988 the GHS identified the causes of long-standing illness. Among children aged 0–15 respiratory disease was by far the most important cause, reported by 7%. This was followed by ear complaints, 2% and skin complaints, 2%. The third national study of morbidity on general practice carried out in 1981–1982 collected the conditions presented at consultations with a general practitioner (GP). These were coded using an adaptation of the International Classification of Diseases (ICD, 1977) as used for coding causes of death[6]. The results for children aged 0–4 and 5–14 are given in the columns on consultations on Table 1.2. Although respiratory diseases accounted for a very small proportion of childhood deaths, they accounted for almost one-third of consultations with GPs. In contrast, injury and poisoning, which are the major cause of death, contributed little to the GP's workload. Diseases of the nervous system and sense organs accounted for 15% of consultations, signs and symptoms for another 10%.[7]

The admissions data in Table 1.2 show comparable information for children's admissions to hospital derived from the 1985 Hospital In-patient Enquiry (HIPE).[8]

About one-fifth of hospital admissions were for diseases of the respiratory system. This was less than for GP consultations. In contrast, injury and poisoning accounted for 1 in 5 admissions for older children and 1 in 10 of those children aged 0–4 years. Whilst cancer was responsible for almost one-quarter of deaths in children aged 5–14, it accounted for only 2% of admissions and an insignificant proportion of GP consultations.

In summary, the data shown in Table 1.2 illustrate the different pictures of children's health which are obtained from different sources of data.

In 1985/1986 OPCS carried out a major survey of disability.[9] Its main aim was to estimate the prevalence of disability arising from physical, mental and sensory causes and to classify it by type and severity. Figure 1.2 summarizes the findings for children. Overall 3% of children were found to have a disability. This is slightly lower than the prevalence of limiting long-standing illness recorded in the GHS (see Fig. 1.1). This is because the disability survey used a large series of questions and a standard threshold level to determine who should be included in the estimates, whereas the GHS relies on the answers to a single question. Figure 1.2 shows that for each age group boys had a higher prevalence of disability than girls. Prevalence was higher in the 5–9 and 10–15 year age groups than in younger children and infants.

Children's disabilities were classified into 11 types: locomotion, reaching and stretching, dexterity, seeing, hearing, personal care, continence, communication, behaviour, intellectual functioning and consciousness. Behavioural disability was the most common — identified in 2% of children. One per cent of children were found to have each of locomotion, continence and intellectual functioning disabilities. The other types of disability were found among fewer than 1% of children. Individual types of disability did not usually

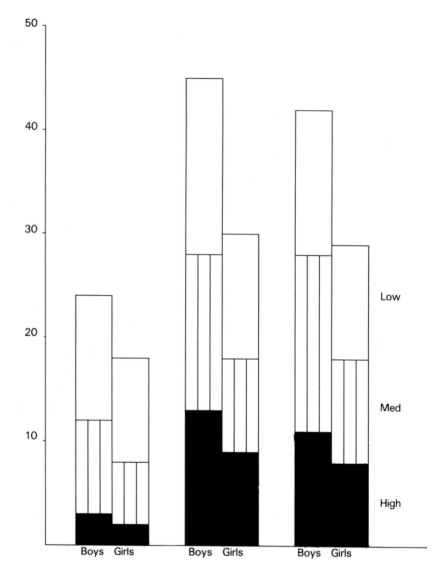

Fig. 1.2 Prevalence of disability. Rate per 1000 children. Data from OPCS survey of disability in Great Britain.[9]

ocur in isolation. The children in the survey had an average of 2.7 of the 11 types of disability identified. So, for example, a child with physical disabilities of locomotion and reaching and stretching may also have a behavioural disability.

OPCS also has regular systems for monitoring the incidence of infectious diseases[10] in childhood and of congenital malformations[11] identified in the first week of life.

Measles notifications decreased following the introduction of immunization in the 1960s from an average of 403 000 per year in 1960–1964 to an average of 170 000 in 1970–1974, and then to 90 000 in 1980–84. In 1988 a combined vaccine for measles, mumps and rubella (MMR) was introduced. The annual total has since decreased to less than 10 000 in 1991. Similarly the numbers of notifications for rubella fell from 25 000 in 1989 to 7000 in 1991. The figures for mumps were 21 000 and 3000. These are quite dramatic changes following a mass public health initiative. Whooping cough vaccine has also become more acceptable to parents over the last 10 years, resulting in only 5000 notifications in 1991 — 34% of the number in 1987.

In contrast the notifications of meningococcal meningitis have been increasing. Between 1977 and 1984 notifications were 450–500 a year. This figure rose to over 1000 in 1990 and 1991. This was the peak of an upsurge similar to that of 1973–1974. Food poisoning has also increased generally during the 1980s, with rates being highest in children under 5 years.

There has been a long-term decrease in all the major types of congenital malformations. For example in 1980, 22 per 10 000 babies were born with central nervous system malformations. As can be seen from Figure 1.3, by 1990 the rate had fallen to 5.1 per 10 000. The rates for cleft lip and/or palate were 13.9 in 1980 and 10.7 in 1990 and for Down's syndrome 7.3 in 1980 and 5.9 in 1990. Using information from notifications of abortion we estimate that only about three-tenths of the reductions in central nervous system abnormalities are due to prenatal detection and abortion. The rates appear to be declining mainly for other reasons.

A series of surveys on dental health carried out by OPCS for the Department of Health includes a standard dental examination. Surveys were carried out on children in 1973 and 1983.[12] Substantial improvements were found in the state of children's teeth at all ages. In 1973 15-year-olds had an average of 7 filled teeth. This average had fallen to 5 in 1983. (The survey is being repeated in 1993.)

Table 1.3 Percentages of children using health services

Service used	Age (years)	Boys	Girls	All children
GP in last 2 weeks	0–4	26%	22%	24%
	5–15	10%	13%	12%
Outpatients/casualty	0–4	14%	10%	12%
in last 3 months	5–15	11%	9%	10%
Inpatient in last year	0–4	12%	8%	10%
	5–15	7%	6%	7%

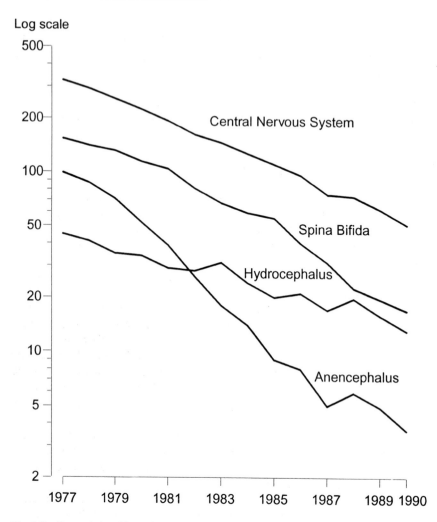

Log scale

Fig. 1.3 Congenital malformations. Rates per 100 000 births for selected conditions in England and Wales. Data from OPCS.[11]

USE OF HEALTH SERVICES

As well as asking questions about health status, the GHS also each year asks parents about the use of GP and hospital services by their children. The results for 1990 are summarized in Table 1.3. Almost one-quarter of children under 5 had consulted the GP in the 2 weeks prior to interview. This represents an average of 8 consultations per year for each child under 5. The proportions consulting and the average number of consultations per year halved for older children. Both these measures of contact with GPs had generally doubled since the survey began in 1972. This was not true for contacts with hospital services.

In 1990 just over one-tenth of children had been to outpatients or casualty in the 3 months before interview. This represents about 70 contacts per 100 children per year. These figures are only slightly higher than those for 1972. The proportion of children who had been inpatients in the year before interview decreased among the under 5s but not among older children. Nevertheless, 10% of under 5s and 7% of older children had been in hospital in the previous year. This is equivalent to 14 and 8 stays per 100 children aged 0–4 and 5–15 respectively.

HEALTH-RELATED BEHAVIOUR

The importance of monitoring health-related behaviour has been emphasized by 'The Health of the Nation'.[13] This strategy for health sets out targets to be reached in future years. As well as target mortality and morbidity rates, two targets were set for children's health-related behaviour. The first of these relates to smoking.

OPCS has carried out a survey of secondary schoolchildren's smoking every other year since 1982. In the early surveys girls and boys had similar smoking behaviour. But in 1986 and subsequent surveys, girls were found to be slightly more likely to smoke than boys. For example, in 1986 7% of boys were regular smokers compared with 12% of girls — 10% of all children aged 11–15 years. This prevalence rate fell to 8% in 1988. The 'Health of the Nation' target was based on 1988 and suggested that smoking prevalence should reduce by 33% by 1994. The 1990 survey,[14] however, showed a small, but not statistically significant, rise in regular smoking among secondary school children to 10%.

The 1990 children's smoking survey also included questions about drinking. Forty per cent of children aged 11–15 in England said they never drank alcohol, but 13% drank at least once a week. For children aged 15, this figure was almost one-quarter.

Nutrition is a particularly difficult subject on which to collect population-based information. However OPCS has carried out a survey of the mothers of newborn babies every 5 years since 1975.[15] Whether or not babies were breast-fed at all is a simple measure of infant feeding practice, although the surveys collected many more details. In 1975 only 51% of babies in England and Wales were breast-fed at all. After substantial education campaigns aimed at parents and professionals, this incidence rose to 67% in 1980. However both the 1985 and 1990 surveys showed no further increase in breast-feeding. OPCS is now carrying out a detailed survey of toddlers' diets which will enhance knowledge in this area.

The Second 'Health of the Nation' target relating to children is in the sexual health area. It is to reduce by at least 50% the conception rate among girls under 16 by the year 2000 from the 1989 baseline. OPCS is able to calculate conception rates by summing live and stillbirths and legal abortions lagged back to age at conception. Spontaneous miscarriages are not recorded and so not included in this conception rate but are believed to be fairly constant from year to year. Between 1980 and 1989 the conception rate for under-14-year olds, 14- and 15-year-olds increased to reach 0.9, 6.0 and 20.7 conceptions per 1000 girls in each age group respectively. The first year of monitoring this target, 1990, showed a further increase to rates of 1.3, 6.6 and 21.6 per 1000.[16]

SOCIOECONOMIC DIFFERENCES IN CHILDREN'S HEALTH

Socioeconomic differences in infant and childhood mortality were reviewed for the years 1979–1980, 1982–1983, and published as part of the Registrar General's decennial supplement series.[17] Some similar analyses on infant and perinatal mortality are published each year.[18] In addition the GHS and other surveys publish analyses by socioeconomic groups. In general, for the indicators discussed in this paper, there is a linear relationship with socioeconomic status. So, for example, fewer than 5% of babies born into families where the father is in social class I (professional) have a low birth weight (less than 2.5 kg). This proportion rises steadily through the social classes to almost 8% in social class V (unskilled). The infant mortality rate varies in the same way. For example, in 1990, looking at births within marriage where husband's occupation can be coded, the infant mortality rate in social class I was 5.6 per 1000 live births, rising to 11.2 in social class V. The group where occupation could not be classified also had a high rate — 10.5 per 1000 live births. Death rates among older children follow the same pattern, with the social class gradient for deaths from injury and poisoning being particularly large.

For morbidity the picture is not so consistent. But the GHS identifies for boys and, to a lesser extent, girls, the expected higher prevalence of limiting long-standing illness among the lower (manual) socioeconomic groups. The 1982 morbidity study in general practice[19] shows the expected differences for infectious disease, respiratory and digestive system diseases, symptoms and ill-defined conditions and accidents, injury and poisoning.

Socioeconomic status is not available from the surveys of schoolchildren's smoking and drinking carried out by OPCS. However, the infant feeding surveys show striking differences in breast-feeding by social class. At 6 weeks about 70% of babies in social class I are still being breast-fed. This falls to about 20% of those in social class V and is even lower for babies in lone mother families. This suggests that there may be considerable socioeconomic variations in other health-related behaviours, as there are in adults.

KEY POINTS FOR CLINICAL PRACTICE

This chapter shows how we can use the considerable amount of routinely collected information to monitor children's health. For the past 10 years it has shown:

Mortality

- Continuing improvements for all groups of children for all the main causes of death.

Morbidity

- There is possibly more long-standing illness and no decline in short-term illness.
- There are fewer congenital malformations in newborn babies.
- The incidence of major childhood infectious diseases is decreasing.

Health-related behaviour

- Patterns of infant feeding are not changing.
- The decline in children's smoking prevalence during the 1980s may have halted.
- Conceptions to girls under 16 continue to increase.

Variations

- Considerable differences in mortality, morbidity and health-related behaviour continue between boys and girls and between children from different socioeconomic groups.

REFERENCES

1 Dunnell K. Monitoring children's health. Population Trends 60. London: HMSO. 1990
2 Mortality statistics, general, series DH1. London: HMSO (annual publication)
3 Mortality statistics, cause, series DH2. London: HMSO (annual publication)
4 Mortality statistics, childhood, series DH6. London: (annual publication)
5 General household survey. London: HMSO (annual publication)
6 International Classification of Diseases 1975, Volume 1. HMSO. 1977
7 Morbidity statistics in general practice 1981–82, series MB5 no.1. London: HMSO. 1986
8 Department of Health and Social Security and Office of Population Censuses and Surveys. Hospital In-Patient Enquiry 1985. London: HMSO. 1987
9 Bone M, Meltzer H. The prevalence of disability among children. London: HMSO. 1989
10 Communicable disease statistics, series MB2. London HMSO: (annual publication)
11 Congenital malformation statistics, series MB3. London HMSO: (annual publication)
12 Todd J, Dodd T. Children's dental health in the United Kingdom 1983. London: HMSO. 1985
13 The Health of the Nation, a strategy for health in England. London: HMSO. 1992
14 Lader D, Matheson J. Smoking among secondary school children 1990. London: HMSO. 1991
15 White A, Freeth S, O'Brien M. Infant feeding 1990. London: HMSO. 1992
16 Conception statistics 1990. Population Trends 69. London: HMSO. 1992
17 Occupational mortality, childhood supplement, series DS8. London: HMSO. 1988
18 Mortality statistics, perinatal and infant: social and biological factors. London: HMSO. 1992
19 Morbidity statistics from general practice 1981–82: socioeconomic analyses, series MB5 no. 2. London: HMSO. 1990

2

Medicolegal reports about children

F. N. Bamford

FOR THE BENEFIT OF CHILDREN

The provision of reports for medicolegal purposes is an important part of paediatric practice. Courts rely on them in reaching decisions which often have far-reaching effects on the lives of children. The reports are, therefore, for the benefit of children and this should be foremost in the thoughts of those who prepare them.

They may be requested in a variety of circumstances, usually one of the following:

1. When an offence against a child has been committed or is suspected.
2. When a child needs or is thought to need protection.
3. When decisions have to be made about future care, for example custody and contact in private law proceedings or in relation to fostering and adoption.
4. When damages are being claimed on behalf of children in cases of accident or medical negligence.

This chapter is mostly concerned with reports relating to child protection and family proceedings.

WHO ASKS FOR REPORTS?

Statements may be requested by police officers or social workers from paediatricians or junior staff responsible for the initial care of abused children. They are entitled to expect a prompt response to enable them to carry out their duties efficiently.

Reports may also be commissioned by solicitors to help them in the defence of clients charged with criminal offences against children or in the representation of children or other parties to family or adoption proceedings, or in anticipation of a possible action for damages. In these circumstances, solicitors usually approach a senior paediatrician known to them, or one from a list kept by the Law Society of medical practitioners willing to give expert testimony or an acknowledged expert in an area of practice relevant to the case.

FORMAT

There are four ways in which information and opinion can be presented:

1. In statements to the police which may later be used in the prosecution of crime it is obligatory to use a standard Criminal Justice Act form (Fig. 2.1).

2. For proceedings in the High Court, for example, in wardship, or in family proceedings, reports are most conveniently presented in affidavit form (Fig. 2.2).

3. A less formal medical report is appropriate when an opinion is requested and it is uncertain whether there will be legal proceedings (Fig. 2.3). The purpose of reports should always be stated and, if necessary, they can be exhibited with sworn affidavits at a later stage.

4. In specific circumstances, for example an adoption application, the medical report may be set out in a form designed for the purpose (Fig. 2.4).

Date, signature and declaration of truth

In the early stages of a child abuse inquiry it is often uncertain whether the statement will be used in legal proceedings but it is wise to presume that it will be used and to prepare it accordingly. In family proceedings the rules require that statements are dated, signed and include a declaration of truth and the understanding that they may be placed before the Courts.

They are now prefaced by the following:

> I make the following statement of x pages believing it to be true and I understand that it may be placed before the Court in connection with proceedings under the Childen Act, 1989.

Identification

After the initial declaration, statements should set out the qualifications, professional appointments and any special experience of the person making the statement. A lengthy curriculum vitae is not required. All that is needed is a brief paragraph giving the Court an indication of the expertise of the witness.

Origin and basis of the report

Identification should be followed by a paragraph stating who requested the report. It may be the local authority, a solicitor instructed by a parent, relative or foster parent, or a solicitor acting for the child on the instruction of a guardian-ad-litem. Exceptionally a report may be commissioned by a Court from an expert agreed by the parties to the proceedings.

Reports may be based either on examinations of children and interviews with their parents or simply on consideration of the clinical records or reports

C.I.D. 9.

BARSETSHIRE CONSTABULARY

STATEMENT OF WITNESS

(Criminal Justice Act, 1967, ss. 2, 9; M.C. Act 1980, s. 102; M.C. Rules 1981, r.70)

STATEMENT OF...

Age of witness (if over 21 enter 'over 21')..

Occupation of witness..

Address...

....

This statement (consisting of ...... pages each signed by me) is true to the best of my knowledge and belief and I make it knowing that, if it is tendered in evidence, I shall be liable to prosecution if I have wilfully stated in it anything which I know to be false or do not believe to be true.

Dated the.. day of ...., 19........

(Signed).........................

Statement taken by:

....

on........................

Fig. 2.1   First page of standard form for statements to the police.

IN THE HIGH COURT OF JUSTICE

FAMILY DIVISION

BARCHESTER DISTRICT REGISTRY

IN THE MATTER OF

            HENRY GRANTLY

            –and–

IN THE MATTER OF

            THE CHILDREN ACT, 1989

BETWEEN

            BARSETSHIRE COUNTY COUNCIL   <u>Applicant</u>

            –and–

            THEOPHILUS GRANTLY

            –and–

            SUSAN GRANTLY   <u>Respondents</u>

REPORT AND OPINION OF DR. JOHN BOLD

I John Bold will say as follows:

1.   My professional qualifications are:
      Doctor of Medicine, Member of the Royal College of Physicians.
      I am a Consultant Paediatrician attending Hiram's Hospital,
      Barchester.

2.   The following report was requested by Messrs. Cox and Cumming,
      Solicitors acting for the defendants. It is based on an
      examination of the minor at the Health Centre, Plumstead
      ....

Fig. 2.2   First page of standard layout for an affidavit.

DEPARTMENT OF PAEDIATRICS
BARCHESTER GENERAL HOSPITAL
BARCHESTER

MEDICAL REPORT ON:

MARY JONES

in connection with family proceedings.

I make the following statement of x pages believing it to be true
and I understand that it may be placed before the Court in
connection with proceedings under the Children Act, 1989.

signed ....

Date   ....

1.   The following report was requested by Messrs. Finney's
      Solicitors acting for the County Council. It is based
      on ....

Fig. 2.3 Recommended opening layout of medical report in case of suspected child abuse.

PRIVATE AND CONFIDENTIAL   **FORM C**

Agency ....

Address.. Social Worker ....

.... Telephone..

Medical Adviser .... Telephone..

If any problems arise in completing this form, please contact the Medical Adviser. Refer to attached sheets if space is inadequate.

MEDICAL REPORT & DEVELOPMENTAL ASSESSMENT OF CHILD UNDER 5 YEARS REFERRED FOR ADOPTION OR RECEIVED INTO CARE
Please complete only sections 1–6 on pages 1–3

Child's surname .... Forename(s)... M/F

Also known as .... Date of birth .... Ref. no....................

Date of examination.. Age at examination...

IMPORTANT *The following information should be available to the doctor making the examination*

Any previous medical report   *Family history of parents*
Neo-natal report/Obstetric report   *List of placements/caregivers*
Medical history (inc record of immunisations)   *List of nurseries etc*
Growth charts to date   *Any relevant specialist reports*
THE CHILD SHOULD BE ACCOMPANIED BY ITS CURRENT CAREGIVER

1. Summary by examining doctor or medical adviser of anything in the collected information which is likely to be relevant to the child's present condition or future prospects *(eg genetic conditions in family; obstetric or neonatal complications; disability; previous illness, accidents and operations; history of growth, development, speech and learning; frequent changes of caregiver etc.)*

2. Is the child attending hospital, clinic or other special unit or receiving medication or other treatment?

3. Comments from current caregiver on child's well-being and behaviour
(Please give name of caregiver. Indicate if current caregiver is not present)

Fig. 2.4 First page of standard form for medical report for adoption of child under the age of 5 years. This form is produced by the British Agencies for Adoption and Fostering (BAAF) Medical Group.

of others. This should be stated and it is particularly important to record the date of any examination because findings may change with time.

RESTRICTION OF EXAMINATIONS

There is a presumption that examinations of children for the purpose of adducing evidence in legal proceedings are potentially damaging to them. They should be avoided if possible. In criminal cases a balance has to be struck between the requirements of justice and the welfare of children. Repeated examinations in connection with claims for damage are inevitable but not usually intrusive.

In family proceedings there are statutory restrictions. No person may cause a child to be medically or psychiatrically examined or otherwise assessed for the preparation of expert evidence for use in proceedings without leave of the Court.[2] The same applies to wardship proceedings in the High Court. Paediatricians called upon to give second opinions for legal purposes should be careful not to examine children unless they have a copy of a Court order permitting them to do so.

DISCLOSURE OF RECORDS

Children, any persons authorized to act for them, or any persons with parental responsibility may apply to the holders of medical records for access to them and, with certain exceptions, it must be given.[3] Complete sets of notes and documents can be obtained to assist in the preparation of reports. Those documents considered should be listed in the report.

HEARSAY

What is required in a report is observation of fact and a medical opinion. Since the cornerstone of medical diagnosis is the history there can be problems with the rules of evidence and in particular with the use of hearsay. In criminal cases the rules will be strictly applied and hearsay should be kept out of reports. In civil proceedings before the High Court or a County Court and in family proceedings in a Magistrates' Court 'evidence in connection with the upbringing maintenance or welfare of a child' is admissible notwithstanding any rules of law relating to hearsay.[4] Wardship proceedings in the High Court amount to an investigation rather than an adversarial contest and the strict rules of evidence do not apply.[5]

RELEVANT EVIDENCE

In writing a report the facts and observations on which the final opinion depends should be set out first. There are two ways to do this. The first is to use the normal medical method of recording the complaint, history of illness, previous health, development, family medical history etc. followed by the observations on examination. Alternatively, in complex cases when there are several issues, it may be better to write a medical chronology commencing at conception and leading to the final examination.

Evidence should be included only if it is relevant, i.e. it has a logical relationship to the opinion that is reached or the matter requiring proof. If evidence is insufficiently relevant it may be inadmissible.

In each type of report, except for those on preprinted examination forms, it is useful to number the paragraphs. This makes it easier for lawyers to refer to specific parts of the report, for example, during cross-examination.

MEDICAL OPINION

The report should conclude with a medical opinion. Opinions on various issues relevant to the case should be enumerated. Not all opinions can be given with confidence and there should be some indication of the degree of certainty including, if appropriate, references to the medical literature. Copies are often attached to reports and are helpful. Likewise, growth charts and photographs can be attached as exhibits to reports.

AMENDMENTS AND SUPPLEMENTARY REPORTS

It is important to take great care in preparation because once a report has been filed or served in family proceedings it may not be amended without leave of the Court. This has to be requested in writing and it can be the subject of representations by parties not wishing it to be amended.[6] Supplementary statements can be filed provided that they are within any time limits specified by the Court.

TIMING

One of the fundamental aims of the Children Act, 1989 is to avoid delay. The Act makes it clear that delay in Court proceedings is generally harmful to children and should be avoided.[7] In family proceedings the Court has to 'draw up a timetable with a view to determining the question without delay'; and 'give such directions as it considers appropriate for the purpose of ensuring, so far as is reasonably practicable, that that timetable is adhered to'.[8] It follows that reports have to be provided promptly and they must be filed before the hearing. Unless a strict timetable has been defined by the Court, the rule applying to wardship, that they should be served on the other parties at least 2 weeks ahead of the hearing, is a reasonable objective.

DISCLOSURE

Medical reports in family proceedings are confidential. Normal practice is to send them to the instructing solicitors and leave it to them to serve them on the other parties. As a matter of professional courtesy one may wish to disclose the report to colleagues especially if the issues or findings are contentious. It is sometimes helpful to Courts to receive an agreed medical opinion but disclosure without leave of the Court except to parties to the proceedings and their legal representatives is illegal.[9] Reports can be disclosed to guardians-ad-litem and welfare officers and in wardship proceedings paediatricians have a positive duty to cooperate with guardians.

Reports should be objective and not partisan. Sometimes they are not helpful and may even be damaging to the case of the instructing solicitor's client. In criminal proceedings they will not be disclosed but in family proceedings failure to disclose is contrary to the spirit of the Children Act and it does not often happen. An unfavourable report may result in the paediatrician being called to give evidence by an opposing lawyer.

The legal professional privilege allowing concealment of evidence can be overridden in wardship. Production of a medical report from a potential expert witness, not called to give evidence by the party for whom it was prepared, can be required.[10] In most cases all parties to proceedings are aware of reports that are commissioned and if they are not produced, deductions are drawn about their content. However, Courts do not have power in proceedings under the Children Act, 1989, as they have in Wardship, to override legal privilege with respect to the disclosure of medical reports.[11]

SWEARING AFFIDAVITS

Reports are often submitted as sworn affidavits. This means that the truth of their content has been attested before an approved solicitor or Commissioner for Oaths. The fact that an affidavit has been provided does not exonerate the person swearing it from attending for cross-examination and if he or she fails to attend the affidavit cannot be used.

CONCLUSION

Well-produced and well-reasoned reports are a means by which Courts can be influenced and their powers and resources harnessed for children. This applies particularly to wardship, private law and family proceedings, and to a lesser extent to criminal and other proceedings. Almost all lawyers are sympathetic to these aims but have an overriding professional obligation to their clients. However, Family Proceedings courts have a duty to put the welfare of children before all else and in this respect, paediatricians have a common purpose.

KEY POINTS FOR CLINICAL PRACTICE

- Courts rely on medical reports in reaching decisions which often have far-reaching effects on the lives of children. The reports are, therefore, for

the benefit of children and this should be foremost in the thoughts of those who prepare them.
- In cases of child abuse, statements may be required by police officers or social workers, who are entitled to expect a prompt response to enable them to carry out their duties efficiently.
- In criminal cases the rules of evidence apply, and hearsay must be kept out of reports; in civil proceedings which concern the welfare of a child, hearsay evidence may be permissible.
- Reports should be objective and not partisan.

REFERENCES

1 Family Proceedings Court (Children Act, 1989) Rules, 1991, Rule 17
2 Family Proceedings Court (Children Act, 1989) Rules, 1991, Rule 18
3 Access to Health Records Act, 1990
4 The Children (Admissibility of Hearsay Evidence) Order, 1991
5 Re E (a Minor) Wardship (1984) WLR 156 at 159
6 Family Proceedings Court (Children Act, 1989) Rules, 1991, Rule 19
7 An Introduction to the Children Act, 1989. Department of Health. London: HMSO, 1989: p. 3
8 The Children Act, 1989, Section 11. London: HMSO
9 Family Proceedings Court (Children Act, 1989) Rules, 1991, Rule 23
10 Re A (Minors) (Disclosure of Material) 1991. Family Law p 476
11 Re B (Minors) (Disclosure of Medical Reports). Times Law Report 29th March, 1993

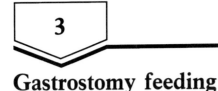

3

Gastrostomy feeding

J. E. Grunow   P. Chait   S. Savoie   C. Mullan   P. Pencharz

Normal healthy children who are provided with a proper diet will voluntarily eat enough food to meet their nutritional needs. Illness, however, renders some children incapable of meeting their nutrient requirements through voluntary oral intake. Children in a prolonged comatose state have no cognitive control of eating. Many children with oral–motor dysfunction from cerebral palsy or trauma cannot maintain normal nutrition. Some children with chronic disease such as cystic fibrosis cannot voluntarily eat enough food to compensate for the nutrient losses and metabolic demands imposed by their disease.[1]

Children whose illness limits their voluntary oral intake can be nourished properly using involuntary enteral feeding techniques. Nasogastric or nasojejunal feeding tubes are effective delivery systems for patients whose nutritional rehabilitation or supplementation period will be no longer than 6–8 weeks. However, whenever it becomes apparent that involuntary feeding will be necessary for a longer period, a permanent feeding tube, such as a gastrostomy, should be inserted.

Before 1980 the only approach to gastrostomy placement was surgical. In 1980 Gauderer et al[2] described gastrostomy placement by a percutaneous endoscopic technique. A radiologically guided antegrade technique[3] was described a few years later, followed by the more popular retrograde technique.[4] These new approaches to placement have proven to be cost-effective and have demonstrated morbidity and mortality rates comparable to those of the operative approach.[4,5] Consequently, the options for gastrostomy placement now include endoscopic and radiological approaches, through percutaneous techniques, as well as the surgical approach.

Development of these percutaneous techniques has renewed interest in the use of gastrostomies as a method of providing enteral nutritional support. There has been a concomitant growth in the variety of replacement tubes and in enteral feeding formulas. This has facilitated nutrition support on an ambulatory basis, using pump-regulated overnight enteral feeding technology. Currently in the Home Feeding Program at The Hospital for Sick Children, Toronto, we have 180–200 patients on overnight enteral feeds compared with 8–12 on total parenteral nutrition (TPN). This type of care is best delivered by a Nutrition Support Team, involving dietetic, medical and nursing members. The authors of this chapter represent all of the health care disciplines involved at The Hospital for Sick Children. Dr Grunow was on sabbatical leave at The Hospital for Sick Children during 1991–1992; his experience with percutaneous endoscopic gastrostomies at the Children's Hospital of Oklahoma is included to provide the reader with a full picture of recent advances in this area.

PERCUTANEOUS GASTROSTOMY TECHNIQUES

The necessity for a gastrostomy is evaluated by the referring physician in consultation with the paediatrician, paediatric gastroenterologist or physician in clinical nutrition. Once it has been decided to carry out a gastrostomy, the decision on an operative or percutaneous technique is made. The percutaneous techniques are contraindicated only when the liver or transverse colon is positioned directly over the proposed gastrostomy site. The efficacy and safety of these techniques have been clearly established,[4,5] and they are the procedure of choice for some high-risk patients.[5] Thus we use the percutaneous approach primarily and reserve operative gastrostomy for patients whose illness requires antireflux surgery in addition to a gastrostomy.

Percutaneous endoscopic gastrostomy

Patients referred for percutaneous endoscopic gastrostomy are seen first in the clinic for a complete medical evaluation and laboratory assessment of clotting function. They are admitted the morning of the procedure, at which time informed consent is obtained and an intravenous infusion (IV) is started. The procedure is performed in an endoscopy suite, but we have performed it easily in the intensive care unit or even in the patient's room when necessary.

Although the percutaneous endoscopic gastrostomy can be done under general anaesthesia, we typically use intravenous sedation: meperidine 2 mg/kg plus either diazepam 0.2 mg/kg or midazolam 0.1 mg/kg. Patients are carefully monitored with continuous electrocardiogram (ECG) and pulse oximetry. Cefazolin sodium (30mg/kg) is given before the procedure.

The gastrostomy site is localized endoscopically as the point of brightest transillumination through the stomach on to the anterior abdominal wall. Failure to identify this point of maximal brightness implies that the transverse colon or liver is anterior to the stomach, a contraindication to proceeding with percutaneous endoscopic gastrostomy. The skin at this location is prepared and anaesthetized with 1% lignocaine.

The stomach is inflated to bring it close to the abdominal wall and push the colon downward. Through the point of maximal brightness, a 20-gauge needle with stylet is introduced into the stomach under endoscopic visualization. A wire guide ('push' technique) or suture ('pull' technique) is threaded through the neeedle into the stomach, snared by the endoscopist and pulled out of the mouth with the gastroscope.

In the 'push' technique, a tapered gastrostomy tube is threaded over the wire guide at the mouth end and pushed until it emerges through the abdominal wall. In the 'pull' technique, the mouth end of the suture is tied to a tapered gastrostomy tube and the abdominal end of the suture is pulled until the tube is pulled through the abdominal wall.

A disc or T-bar on the internal end of the tube prevents external tube migration, and a similar disc or T-bar passed over the external end fits against the abdominal wall and prevents internal tube migration. The stomach and abdominal wall are kept in close approximation by this mechanism until adhesions form.

Patients recover in their room after the procedure with the following orders:

1. Gastrostomy tube straight drainage for 24 h
2. Nil per os or gastrostomy tube for 24 h
3. IV at maintenance
4. Observations of temperature, pulse, respiration and blood pressure every 30 min × 2 and 2 hourly × 2
5. Analgesia — meperidine/paracetamol 4-hourly
6. Antibiotics — cefazolin 30 mg/kg every 6 h × 2

The following day, readiness to feed is assessed by the volume of gastrostomy drainage and the presence of abdominal distention. A soft, non-distended abdomen and gastric drainage less than 30–50 ml every 8 h indicate adequate gastric emptying function, and imply that the patient will tolerate feedings. Patients are discharged when feedings are well-tolerated, usually 2–3 days after the procedure. They are seen 1 week after discharge to assess tube function and gastrostomy site. The gastrostomy tube is not routinely changed; however, after adequate time for adhesion formation (3–6 months) the tube can be safely changed according to patient preference.

Although gastrostomy-related morbidity does not differ from that of operative gastrostomy, the clinician should be aware of two problems that occur with clinically significant frequency. Gastrocolic fistula is reported in 2.2% of percutaneous endoscopic gastrostomies and may be clinically apparent as chronic diarrhoea, especially associated with feedings. Gastro-oesophageal reflux requiring antireflux surgery occurs more frequently (12–33%),[5,6] primarily in neurologically impaired children. Vomiting may begin weeks or months after the procedure and is unexplained by other illnesses. A barium study of the upper gastrointestinal tract demonstrates the pathology in both problems.

Retrograde percutaneous gastrostomy in children

We have been performing retrograde gastrostomies at The Hospital for Sick Children since November, 1990; the total now numbers 185. The patients ranged in age from 3 weeks (corrected 33 weeks' gestation) to 17 years, with a weight range of 1.7–48 kg. Once a decision for gastrostomy has been made, we adhere to a strict preprocedural protocol. The patient is admitted the night before, at which time informed consent is obtained and oral barium given so that the colon is outlined for the procedure. An IV line and a nasogastric tube are placed on the day of the procedure and feedings withheld, as with any surgical procedure. IV antibiotics (cefazolin sodium, 30 mg/kg) are given routinely before the procedure. The procedure is performed in an interventional radiological suite with a C-arm fluoroscopic unit. Anaesthetic and resuscitation equipment is readily available. Ultrasound is performed before the procedure to outline the lower limits of the liver and spleen. Most procedures are performed under sedation, as follows: body weight less than 6 kg, choral hydrate 50–80 mg/kg (orally); 8–30 kg, pentobarbital 3 mg/kg (IV); and greater than 30 kg, diazepam 0.1 mg/kg (IV).

Meperidine hydrochloride (IV) is given for pain control in patients over 8 kg (1 mg/kg). The drugs can be repeated when necessary. In patients in whom there is concern about the airway, the respiratory status, the cardiac status, or in a patient where lack of cooperation is anticipated, general anaesthesia is used, but more often the procedures are performed under local anaesthetic alone.

A specially trained paediatric nurse who forms part of the intervention team constantly monitors the patient by various means, including continuous ECG and pulse oximetry. After the patient has been sedated and immobilized, the liver and spleen are outlined sonographically and the air-filled stomach and barium-filled colon identified fluoroscopically (Fig. 3.1).[3] The preferred site of puncture lateral to the left rectus muscle is prepared and local anaesthetic introduced (1% lignocaine − 0.5 ml/kg). IV glucagon (0.1–0.3 mg) is given to decrease peristalsis.

Materials used include a neonatal retention suture (Cook, Bloomington, IN), 0.018 in and 0.035 in wires, dilator (Coons, Cook) and Seldinger needle, and finally a Cope–Loop catheter (Cook; Fig. 3.2). The site of puncture is identified and the stomach inflated to see whether it extends far enough inferior (Fig. 3.3). A small incision is then made with no. 11 scalpel blade. The puncture is made under fluoroscopic control with a 20-gauge needle loaded with a neonatal retention suture. The position of the needle is confirmed with the introduction of contrast medium (Fig. 3.4). A 0.018 in wire is then introduced through the needle to deposit the retention suture within the stomach (Fig. 3.3). A second puncture is made adjacent to the first with a 19-gauge Seldinger needle. A 0.035 in wire is then introduced via the needle and the needle removed. A Coons dilator lubricated with Muco Catheter (a proprietary brand of lubricant) is introduced over the wire and the tract dilated. A Cope–Loop (Cook) of appropriate size is introduced into the stomach (15 cm, 8–12 French). The position is confirmed with the introduction of contrast and anterior/posterior and lateral screening (Fig. 3.5). A gastrojejunal tube is inserted as a primary catheter if there is a strong history of reflux or some other indication for jejunal feeds. Its insertion requires the

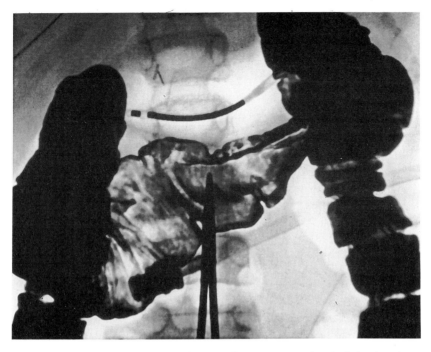

Fig. 3.1 The colon is outlined with barium, a radiopaque nasogastric tube is in place, but the stomach is undistended. This patient was anephric and on peritoneal dialysis; the dialysis catheter is also visible.

introduction of a directional catheter and placement of a wire into the duodenum and then introduction of a gastrojejunal catheter.

Patients are sent directly back to the ward with the following postprocedure orders:

1. Nasogastric and gastrostomy tube straight drainage for 24 h
2. Nil per gastrostomy tube and nasogastric tubes for 24 h
3. IV at maintenance
4. Temperature, pulse, respiration and blood pressure measurement every 15 min × 2, 30 min × 2 and 2-hourly × 2
5. Analgesia — meperdine/paracetamol 4-hourly
6. Antibiotics — further dose if difficult or prolonged procedure
7. Daily dressings

The patients are assessed regularly on the ward by staff of both Radiology and Clinical Nutrition. Orders for feeds and choice of formula are under the control of the Nutrition Team. Patients are usually discharged 3–5 days after the procedure. One week after the procedure they are seen at a gastrostomy tube clinic, at which time the retention suture is cut, tube function assessed, and parents' questions answered. At regular clinic follow-up, the gastrostomy

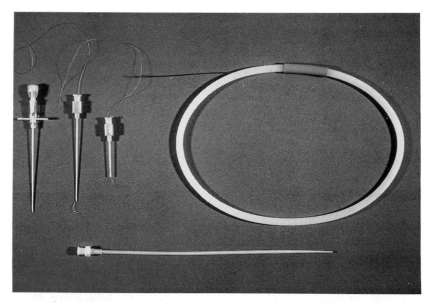

Fig. 3.2 Materials used for the retrograde percutaneous gastrostomy in children. From left to right: Seldinger needle, two sizes of neonatal retention sutures, guide wire (in oval container), and at the bottom a Coons dilator. The Cope-Loop catheter is used as in the gastrostomy tube shown in Figure 3.6.

tube is changed to a balloon-type catheter at 6 weeks, and if indicated to a button at 3 months.

We were unsuccessful in placing the gastrostomy tube in only 2 of the 185 patients; the reason in both cases was gross hepatosplenomegaly. In another patient the tube was misplaced and repositioned during the same procedure. Another patient required laparotomy after the tube was incorrectly placed outside the stomach. Four patients developed mild fever and localized irritation of the peritoneum, a complication that was seen prior to the routine use of preprocedural antibiotics.

GASTROSTOMY MANAGEMENT

Making the decision to have a gastrostomy placed in their child is often difficult for parents.[7] They express concerns about the discomforts their child will experience, the appearance of the tube and their child's ability to eat with the tube in place.[7,8] In our experience, addressing these concerns before the procedure makes it possible for both child and family to adapt better and more quickly. They may find it helpful to meet a family with a child who already has a tube in place. Daily care of the gastrostomy site and tube is the key to minimizing problems. The Nutrition Support nursing team has developed a teaching manual for parents.[9] Teaching begins within a day of tube placement and focuses on gastrostomy site management, the tube, feeding bags, pumps, and tubing.

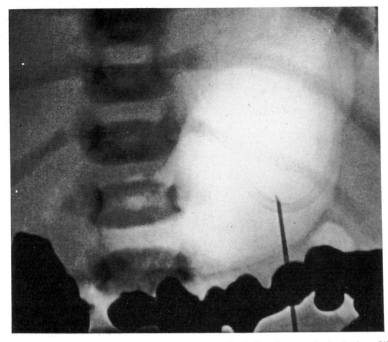

Fig. 3.3 The stomach is shown distended with air, displacing downwards the barium-filled colon. The Seldinger needle is shown about to make the puncture into the distended stomach.

Skin care[10]

Parents are taught to inspect the gastrostomy site daily for signs of inflammation. Under normal circumstances the site is tender and appears red for several days after tube insertion. Thereafter the edges of the site are pink and the tenderness abates. Some form of drainage is common. It may be serosanguineous at first, but typically a light-green or yellow-green purulent discharge predominates. This discharge, which consists of mucus and inflammatory cells, results from the tube rubbing in the tract and may be present in small amounts as long as the gastrostomy is patent. A slight odour is to be expected.

A central concern is how well the gastrostomy tube seals off the tract. The effectiveness of the seal in all types of tubes depends on the fit of the tube within the tract. Tubes with inflatable balloons or moulded mushroom-shaped heads have an additional seal at the gastric end of the tract. The longer (Foley-type) tubes with inflatable balloons have a tendency to rock back and forth and widen the tract, thereby weakening the seal and causing leakage.

Inflammation can be identified through changes observed in the discharge or the skin around the stoma. An increase in the amount of discharge may indicate skin maceration from residual skin moisture or increased irritation of the gastrostomy tract as a result of greater tube mobility. Gastric acid leakage

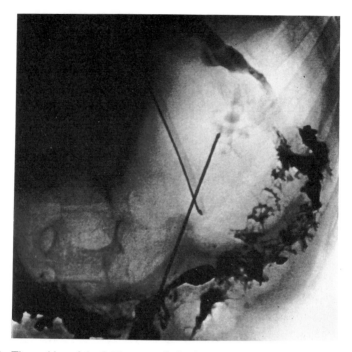

Fig. 3.4   The position of the Seldinger needle in the stomach is confirmed with the injection of contrast medium.

around the tube excoriates the skin, causing it to be red and tender. Infection of the tract or surrounding tissues increases the discharge volume, causing skin induration, tenderness and redness, and imparts a foul odour to the drainage. Usually this can be treated topically. In the rare cases in which the infection is severe enough to cause fever, our experience is that intravenous antibiotics are indicated.

Granulation tissue is usually due to a chemical reaction to the tube. Frequently, there is superimposed secondary infection. Treatment consists of keeping the stoma and surrounding skin as dry and clean as possible. It may be necessary to expose the stoma to air. Rubbing alcohol is useful as a drying agent; although it stings, it is highly effective. Silver nitrate painted on to the granulation tissue may also help. Generally, we have encountered problems with granulation tissue chiefly with the balloon-type catheters and least with the button tubes. Thus it is sometimes necessary to change from one type to the other.

Routine care of the gastrostomy site[11]

The dressing should be changed daily, and the skin washed with mild soap, rinsed and thoroughly dried to prevent maceration. For the first 10 days after

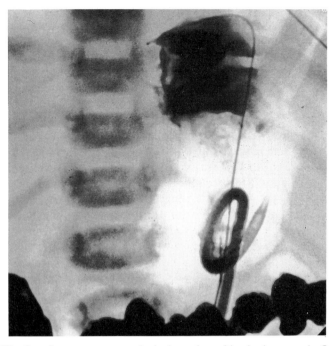

Fig. 3.5 The Cope-Loop gastrostomy tube is shown in position in the stomach. Contrast is seen in the stomach and in the barium-filled colon.

insertion of the tube, patients should refrain from showering or bathing. They may then return to normal activities, including swimming, provided they keep the stoma clean and dry. A thin layer of petroleum jelly protects the skin from the effects of the usual stomal discharge. A barrier cream such as Critic-acid (Sween Corporation, North Mankato, MN, a thick white barrier cream which contains zinc oxide and benzethonium chloride) can be applied to protect the skin when there is an increased discharge of gastric acid. Duoderm (Squibb, Princeton, NJ), a stoma adhesive dressing which has been treated with a colloidal gel of pectin, is used when skin breakdown has occurred. It promotes healing when left in place for a period of time (usually 5–7 days).

The technique used to insert the gastrostomy tube will determine the type of device initially placed. The endoscopically-placed tube has a crossbar (or disc) on the internal side to prevent accidental removal. A similar device fits over the tube on the outside, against the skin. Together, these devices create a sandwich effect with the gastric and abdominal walls in the middle, securing their approximation until sufficient adhesions develop to maintain the integrity of the gastrostomy tract. This type of tube is seldom pulled out inadvertently and is not replaced unless it becomes non-functional. Smaller tubes (12 French and smaller) can be removed by cutting the tube at skin level and pushing the short end into the stomach. If this method is used in a small child or with a larger tube, it may on rare occasions obstruct the bowel at various points, including the pylorus, or even at the ileocaecal valve.

A nephrostomy tube (Fig. 3.6) without an external anchor but secured internally by a pigtail curl is inserted during the radiographic technique. Although it can be left in place for 6–9 months, in some cases it falls out in 2–3 months. Therefore, we have developed a routine whereby the nephrostomy tube is removed at 6–8 weeks and replaced with either a balloon or button-type tube. If a button-type tube is used, the parents are instructed by the nurse specialist how to replace it and are given a spare tube to take home. This routine greatly reduces the need to come to the hospital for tube replacement. Balloon tubes should be inspected daily to determine position. A tube that is not well-secured externally often migrates towards the pylorus and may cause obstruction. Ths migration may also weaken the seal and promote leakage of gastric contents around the tube. Similarly, a poorly inflated or broken internal balloon also allows leaking. Thus, the volume of the inflated balloon (5–7 ml) should be checked weekly.

Replacement tubes

Regardless of the method used to create a gastrostomy, the tube placed during the procedure eventually malfunctions and must be replaced. A trained nurse or physician must carry out the first change. Until recently the primary replacement tube was the Foley-type with an inflatable balloon on the end (Fig. 3.6). The latest versions of these tubes have an external disc to prevent internal migration. Parents can readily be trained to replaced these tubes when the balloon fails, which it does on average every 3–5 months.

Currently, the preferred replacement tube is a device known as the button.[5] It is a mushroom-tipped silicone tube with a shaft length corresponding to the length of the gastrostomy tract, with the external surface flush with the skin (Fig. 3.6). Button tubes with inflatable balloons in the place of the mushroom head are also being produced. Although these are easier to insert, their balloons tend to break after a few months of use. Conversely, the mushroom-type button tube requires an introducer for its insertion but lasts on average 1–2 years. The mushroom tubes are the most stable since they have no external length. They are fitted with an antireflux valve in the tip that prevents leaking through the tube. A special adaptor must be used during feeding to allow the formula to flow through the tube. The button comes with shaft diameters of 18, 24 and 28 French. Each size has three to four shaft lengths varying from 1.2 to 4.4 cm. The appropriate shaft length is determined by measuring the length of the gastrostomy tract, either by using the measuring device supplied with the button or by marking the old gastrostomy tube at skin level before its removal. Once the old tube has been removed, the tract length is measured from the external mark to the top of the balloon or mushroom. It is important that the correct shaft length is used; if it is too long, then leakage will be a problem, and if it is too short, skin

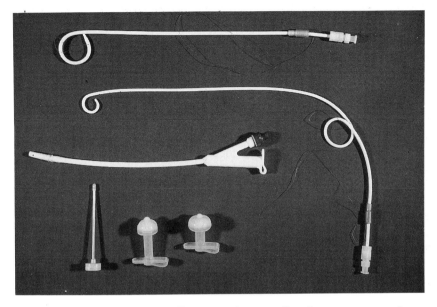

Fig. 3.6 Various gastrostomy tubes. From top to bottom: a Cope-Loop gastrostomy tube; a gastrojejunal tube with a gastric retention loop and a curl at the tip, which with peristalsis maintains the tip in the jejunum; a balloon-type gastrostomy tube (without a retaining disc); two sizes of button gastrostomy tubes plus an introducer.

irritation, pain, and even fissures and abcesses may develop. The button shaft should be rotated daily to ensure that it is freely mobile within the tract and is not migrating out.

The button is an excellent replacement for all patients, except those who require frequent gastric decompression or measurement of residual volume. Most of our patients prefer the appearance and easy maintenance of the button. Buttons should be inserted only by qualified personnel. The tract established with either type of percutaneous gastrostomy insertion is usually smaller than 18 French. It is therefore necessary to dilate the tract in order to insert a button tube. We usually do this by using Foley tubes of increasing external diameter up to 16 French. Parents can do this at home, leaving each size in situ for 7–10 days. Insertion of the button can be uncomfortable for the child, so we routinely administer an oral sedative such as chloral hydrate. Soaking the button in hot water before insertion makes it more pliable and easier to insert. The Bard (Bard Interventional Products, Tewksbury, MA) button comes in a complete kit with an introducer and feeding adaptors.

Formula selection with this tube should exclude liquidized foods, since they may cause the valve to stick in the open position and allow gastric contents to leak. For the same reason, viscous and thick medications should be limited; if they must be used, flushing with soda water after the administration helps minimize valve sticking. The establishment of a nurse specialist gastrostomy clinic has greatly facilitated the routine care of patients. Medical and radiological back-up is always available.

GASTROSTOMY FEEDING

Formulas

The multitude of formulas available for gastrostomy feeding makes it difficult for the clinician to choose the best product to meet each patient's individual requirements. The selection process can be made easier by remembering that all formulas fit into four basic categories: home-liquidized, polymeric, elemental and modular. The following discussion describes the composition of each type and reviews indications for their use. (It does not deal with infant formulas.)

Home-liquidized formulas

Before the evolution of commercial formulas, tube feedings consisted of liquidized whole foods thinned with liquids to allow passage through a fine-bore tube (Table 3.1). Since this food differs from a normal diet only in

Table 3.1   Constituents of enteral formula

	Protein	Fat	Carbohydrate
Home-liquidized*	Whole protein	Long chain triglycerides	Starch, di and monosaccharides
Polymeric*	Whole protein (11–25%)	Long and/or medium chain triglycerides, mono- and diglycerides, lecithin (21–39%)	Starch, maltodextrins, poly-, oligo- and disaccharides (46–66%)
Elemental	Hydrolysed protein, peptides, free amino acids (8–18%)	Long and/or medium chain triglycerides (1–36%)	Starch, maltodextrins poly-, oligo-, di- and monosaccharides (51–91%)
Protein modules	Whole protein, amino acids		
Carbohydrate modules			Glucose polymers, maltodextrins
Fat modules		Long and medium chain triglycerides, lecithin	

*May contain fibre
Figures in brackets indicate percentage of calories.
Adapted from MacBurney et al.[12]

texture, patients with conditions requiring predigested nutrients may not tolerate it, or it may not meet their nutritional requirements. Home-liquidized foods offer some advantages: they cost less than formula food, their composition can be easily altered, micronutrient deficiencies may be avoided, soluble and insoluble fibres may be present, and using home-prepared feeding offers a psychological benefit. On the other hand, the viscosity of the formula may be too thick for the feeding tube, there is greater potential for bacterial contamination, it is difficult to assess actual nutrients received and food preparation is time-consuming. Generally the disadvantages, especially that of contamination, outweigh the advantages, and so the use of home-liquidized feeds is not encouraged.

Polymeric formulas

The name polymeric refers to the fact that the protein, fat and carbohydrate components of these formulas are mostly in non-hydrolysed forms (i.e. whole protein, mainly long chain triglycerides (LCTs), starch and glucose polymers). The formulas are designed for patients with no gastrointestinal problems that would significantly impair nutrient digestion and absorption.

Polymeric formulas contain between 11 and 25% of total calories in the form of whole proteins of high quality. The quality of a protein is determined by its digestibility and its capacity to support the growth of experimental animals. The protein efficiency ratio is a method of measuring protein quality based on growth of experimental animals in relation to grams of protein consumed. A protein with suboptimal levels of one or more essential amino acids would be required in greater amounts in order to support growth.[13] High-quality protein sources used in formulas include beef, egg white solids, soy protein isolates, casein isolates, lactalbumin, whey, non-fat and whole dry milk, sodium and calcium caseinates.[12]

Polymeric formulas contain between 20 and 40% of total calories as fat. This level is based on the 38% level of fat normally consumed in the average North American diet and the recommendation that it be reduced to 30% of total calories.[14] Sources of fat include long chain triglycerides (butterfat, corn, soy, safflower and sunflower oils), medium chain triglycerides (MCTs; fractionated coconut oil), lecithin, di- and monoglycerides.[12] LCTs serve as a source of concentrated calories (9.0 versus 4.0 kcal/g for protein and carbohydrate) and essential fatty acids and as a carrier of fat-soluble vitamins. They also contribute positive to the 'mouth-feel' and palatability of formulas. MCTs are added to polymeric formulas because of their easy digestion and rapid absorption compared with LCTs.[15]

Carbohydrate is an easily digested and absorbed component of polymeric formulas, providing 46–66% of total calories. Its sources are primarily starch and partially hydrolysed starch.[12] The longer the chain length, the less the contribution to osmolality. Partially hydrolysed starch (maltodextrins, oligo- and polysaccharides) is more soluble and absorbed as rapidly as glucose itself.[16]

Disaccharides in formulas include byproducts of partial starch hydrolysis as well as lactose from milk and sucrose. Lactose and sucrose are contraindicated in cases of primary or secondary disaccharide deficiency as well as in some metabolic conditions. Glucose is generally not present in these formulas, since it contributes to higher osmolality and formula intolerance.

Many polymeric formulas contain added fibre in the range of 3.3–13.3 g total dietary fibre per 1000 ml. The fibre source is soy polysaccharide, which consists of 94% insoluble and 6% soluble fibre.[17] Insoluble fibre absorbs water, thereby increasing faecal bulk and reducing faecal transit time. Soluble fibre serves as a substrate for bacterial fermentation and production of short chain fatty acids, which then serve to increase intestinal cell turnover.[18] Theoretically these effects would be of benefit in constipation, diarrhoea, short gut, and gut atrophy; however, the efficacy of using fibre-supplemented formulas has yet to be proven in controlled clinical trials.

Polymeric formulas are also available in 1.5 and 2.0 kcal/ml, with or without higher nitrogen, for patients with high calorie and/or protein requirements for fluid-restricted patients. Since the renal solute load of these formulas is high, there is a danger of dehydration and elevated urea and electrolytes if patients are not monitored closely and given adequate free water. A higher caloric density may also result in slower gastric emptying, which would be undesirable in patients at risk for reflux.[19]

Vitamin and mineral concentrations of all commercial formulas are based on the levels that will meet established requirements when calorie needs are met. Patients receiving low calorie intakes may need additional vitamin and mineral supplements. Ultratrace minerals such as selenium, chromium and molybdenum are now being added to formulas as a result of reports that low concentrations of these have been found in patients on long-term tube feeds or TPN.[20–22] Carnitine and taurine are also being added to some formulas on the premise that, although they can be synthesized, they may not be produced adequately by sick patients.[23,24]

Elemental formulas

Elemental formulas are designed for patients with significant gastrointestinal disorders such as short gut, inflammatory bowel disease, pancreatitis, lymphangiectasia, protein-losing enteropathy, biliary atresia, radiation enteritis and chronic diarrhoea. In general, the protein, carbohydrate and fat are more hydrolysed in comparison with polymeric formulas.

The level of protein in these formulas ranges from 8 to 18% of total calories in various combinations of protein hydrolysates, oligo-, di-, tri-, and tetrapeptides, and amino acids. The best physical form of protein in terms of absorption and physiological benefits remains unclear. Originally it was believed that proteins had to be luminally hydrolysed to free amino acids before absorption could occur. However, jejunal infusion studies have now shown that di- and tripeptides are also absorbed intact and possibly even more rapidly than free amino acids.[25] Nevertheless, our study of children and adolescents with Crohn's disease was unable to show any important differences in amino nitrogen absorption between amino acids and peptides.[26] Of much greater importance in terms of protein utilization is the balance of amino acids or protein quality; in the same study, we showed significantly better nitrogen retention with a higher-quality protein source.[26] Feeds containing peptides have been found to stimulate greater release of gut hormones and growth factors in experimental animals than amino acids alone.[27,28] In general, it appears there is no benefit in using elemental formulas containing strictly amino acids as a protein source compared with whole proteins and peptides. Evidence to support the widespread use of peptide-containing formulas remains insufficient, although there appears to be an absorptive advantage in critically ill patients.[29]

Fat content of elemental formulas differs from that of polymeric formulas in that some contain a much lower percentage of total calories as fat (1–36%) and often the percentage of MCTs is greater. A very low level of LCTs may be indicated in pancreatitis to avoid stimulating secretion of cholecystokinin-pancreozymin in lymphangiectasia to decrease protein loss from the gut, or in LCT-induced hyperlipoproteinemia.[30–32]

The carbohydrate content of elemental formulas ranges from 51 to 91% of total calories, the higher levels replacing fat calories in low-fat formulas. The type of carbohydrate is similar to that of polymeric formulas, with the exception that a few may contain glucose monomers.

Modules

Protein, fat, and carbohydrate modules are available so that formulas can be altered if necessary to meet an individual patient's needs for higher protein, fat, carbohydrate and/or calories. Obviously such alteration will change the percentage of total calories provided from these macronutrients and may also affect patient tolerance.

Formula delivery and tolerance

There are basically three methods of administering formula: bolus, intermittent and continuous.

Bolus feeds are rapidly instilled via syringe over a few minutes. Generally 4–6 feeds per day are required to provide adequate volumes to meet calorie, nutrient and fluid requirements. Disadvantages of this feeding method are the potential for the occurrence of bloating, cramping, nausea, diarrhoea and/or aspiration.

Intermittent feeds are given slowly by gravity drip or pump 4–6 times per day. The rate can be adjusted to the individual patient's tolerance (½–2 h per feed).

Continuous feed may be necessary for patients unable to tolerate large volumes delivered at relatively high infusion rates because of delayed gastric emptying. Continuous overnight feeds may also be used in children over 1 year of age, allowing for intake of solid food and/or freedom of movement during the day.

A significant proportion of the patients requiring gastrostomy feeding are those with spastic quadriplegia. Many of these children also have delayed gastric emptying.[33] which we have shown is clinically helped by using a whey-based formula and avoiding casein-based formulas. We have also shown that the daily energy needs of these patients are often very low.[34] As mentioned above, it is important to select a product that is designed to meet the higher nutrient-to-energy needs of the infant and young child.

KEY POINTS FOR CLINICAL PRACTICE

- A gastrostomy tube should be placed if nutritional rehabilitation or supplementation will require more than 6–8 weeks.
- The percutaneous gastrostomy approach compares favourably with the operative approach and is the one primarily used. Operative gastrostomy is reserved for patients whose illness requires antireflux surgery.
- Daily care of the gastrostomy site and stabilization of the tube are essential to minimize gastrostomy problems. Parent training is the key to daily gastrostomy care.
- The gastrostomy button is the replacement tube preferred by most patients and parents.
- Polymeric formulas will meet the needs of most children who are gastrostomy-fed.
- Elemental formulas are designed for patients with gastrointestinal disorders.

REFERENCES

1 Durie PR, Pencharz PB. Nutrition in cystic fibrosis. Br Med Bull 1992; 48: 823–847
2 Gauderer MWL, Ponsky JL, Izant RJ Jr. Gastrostomy without laparotomy: a percutaneous endoscopic technique. J Pediatr Surg 1980; 15: 872–875
3 Towbin RB, Ball WS, Jr, Bisset GS, III. Percutaneous gastrostomy and percutaneous gastrojejunostomy in children: antegrade approach. Radiology 1988; 168: 473–476
4 King SJ, Chiat PG, Daneman A, Pereira J. Retrograde percutaneous gastrostomy: a prospective study in 57 children. Pediatr Radiol 1993; 23: 23–25
5 Gauderer MWL. Percutaneous endoscopic gastrostomy: a 10-year experience with 220 children. J Pediatr Surg 1991; 26: 288–294
6 Grunow JE, Al-Hafidh AS, Tunell WP. Gastroesophageal reflux following percutaneous endoscopic gastrostomy in children. J Pediatr Surg 1989; 24: 42–45
7 Huddleston KC, Ferraro AR. Preparing families of children wish gastrostomies. Pediatr Nurse 1991; 33: 72–73

8 Alltop SA. Teaching for discharge: gastrostomy tubes. R.N. 1988; 51: 42–46

9 Bertollo-Harrison D. Your child and home gastrostomy feeding, revised The Hospital for Sick Children, Nutrition Support Nursing Team, 1992 [Copies available from Dr. Pencharz, Price $15 (Canadian dollars) each]

10 Irwin M. Managing leaking gastrostomy sites. Am J Nurs 1988; 88: 359–360

11 Johnson S. A safer gastrostomy for the high risk patient. R.N. 1986; 49: 29–33

12 MacBurney MM, Russell C, Young LS. Formulas. In: Rombeau JL, Caldwell MD, eds. Clinical nutrition: enteral and tube feeding, 2nd edn. Philadelphia: Saunders. 1990.

13 Linder MC. Nutrition and metabolism of proteins. In: Linder MC ed. Nutritional biochemistry and metabolism with clinical applications, 2nd edn. New York: Elsevier. 1991.

14 National Research Council. Diet and health. Implications for reducing chronic disease risk. Washington: National Academy. 1989.

15 Holt PR. MCTs: a useful adjunct in nutritional therapy. Gastroenterology 1967; 53: 961–966

16 Jones BJM, Brown BE, Spiller RC, Silk DBA. Energy dense enteral feeds — the use of high molecular weight glucose polymers. JPEN 1981; 5: 567

17 Fredstrom SB, Baglien KS, Lampe JW, Slavin JL. Determination of the fiber content of enteral feedings. JPEN 1991; 15: 450–453

18 Vahouny GV, Cassidy MM. Dietary fiber and intestinal adaptation. In: Vahouny GV, Kritchevsky D, eds. Dietary fiber: basic and clinical aspects. New York: 1986 Plenum.

19 Hunt JN, Smith JL, Jiang CL. Effect of meal volume and energy density on the gastric emptying of carbohydrates. Gastroenterology 1985; 89: 1326–1330

20 Feller AG, Rudman D, Erve PR et al. Subnormal concentrations of serum selenium and plasma carnitine in chronically tube-fed patients. Am J Clin Nutr 1987; 45: 476–483

21 Jeejheeboy KN, Chu C, Errol B et al. Chromium deficiency, glucose intolerance and neuropathy reversed by chromium supplementation in a patient receiving long-term total parenteral nutrition. Am J Clin Nutr 1977; 30: 531–538

22 Abumrad NN, Schneider AJ, Steel D, Rogers LS. Amino acid intolerance during prolonged total parentenal nutrition reversed by molybdate therapy. Am J Clin Nutr 1981; 34: 2551–2559.

23 Geggel HS, Ament ME, Heckenlively JR, Martin DA, Kopple JD. Nutritional requirement for taurine in patients receiving long-term parenteral nutrition. N Engl J Med 1985; 312: 142–146

24 Feller AG, Rudman D, Erve PR et al. Subnormal concentrations of serum selenium and plasma carnitine in chronically tube-fed patients. Am J Clin Nutr 1987; 45: 476–483

25 Silk DBA, Fairclough PD, Park NG et al. A study of the relations between the absorption of amino acids, dipeptides, water and electrolytes in the normal human jejunum. Clin Sci Mol Med 1975; 49: 401–408

20 Vaisman N, Griffiths A, Pencharz P. Comparison of nitrogen utilization of two elemental diets in patients with Crohn's disease. J. Pediatr Gastroenterol Nutr 1988; 7: 84–88

27 Rerat A, Nunes CS, Mendy F, Roger L. Amino acid absorption and production of pancreatic hormones in non-anaesthetized pigs after duodenal infusions of a milk enzymatic hydrolysate or of free amino acids. Br J Nutr 1988; 60: 121–136

28 Sicar B, Johnson LR, Lichtenberger LM. Effect of chemically defined diets on antral and serum gastrin levels in rats. Am J Physiol 1980; 238: G376–G383

29 Meredith JW, Ditesheim JA, Zaloga GP. Visceral protein levels in trauma patients are greater with peptide diet than intact protein diet. J Trauma 1990; 30: 825–829

30 Havala T, Shronts E, Cerra F. Nutritional support in acute pancreatitis. Gastroenterol Clin North Am 1989; 18: 525–540

31 Holt PR. Dietary treatment of protein loss in intestinal lymphangiectasia: the effect of eliminating dietary long chain triglycerides on albumin metabolism in this condition. J Pediatr 1964; 34: 629–635

32 Partin JS, Partin JC, Schubert WK et al. Liver ultrastructure in abetalipoproteinemia: evolution of micronodular cirrhosis. Gastroenterology 1974; 67: 107–118

33 Fried MD, Khoshoo V, Secker DL et al. Decrease of gastric emptying time and episodes of regurgitation in children with spastic quadriplegia fed a whey-based formula. J Pediatr 1992; 120: 569–572

34 Fried MD, Pencharz PB. Energy and nutrient intakes of children with cerebral palsy. J Pediatr 1991; 119: 947–949.

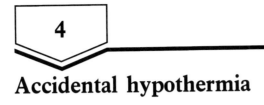

Accidental hypothermia

H. M. Corneli

Accidental hypothermia presents a paradox to the physician. Controlled hypothermia has been used safely in medicine for decades. Case reports of accidental hypothermia have focused on the remarkable survival of occasional victims.[1,2] Large case series[3] have begun to clarify treatment controversies. Yet the same accidents, such as near-drowning or trauma, that occasion the rare hypothermic survival remain the leading causes of childhood death and disability. Accidental hypothermia differs from controlled hypothermia; despite the potential for protection from anoxia, many complications worsen rather than improve the patient's prognosis.

Accidental hypothermia may cause a potentially salvageable patient to appear lifeless; it also complicates treatment, altering some of the fundamental practices of resuscitation. Pediatricians should be familiar with the changes in physiology, diagnosis and management incurred by hypothermia. Methods of patient rewarming, long the subject of debate, can now be evaluated and categorized more objectively. Yet with the recognition that hypothermia is detrimental to most patients, pediatricians must also renew their commitment to prevention.

This paper will not discuss induced hypothermia, perioperative hypothermia, or neonatal hypothermia per se, nor will it encompass cold injuries such as pernio or frostbite.

AETIOLOGY

Defined as a core temperature below 35°C, hypothermia may be occasioned by any marked decrease in heat production or increase in heat loss (Table 4.1). Children are at special risk for accidental hypothermia because of their increased surface-area-to-mass ratio and decreased fat insulation. The newborn is well-known to be at risk; as in the elderly, infants may insidiously become hypothermic due to inadequate residential heating. At later ages children are exposed to events, especially traumatic injury and cold immersion, that may induce hypothermia. The growing popularity of hill-walking, skiing, and other outdoor pursuits will expose an increasing population of children to the risk of accidental hypothermia.

41

Table 4.1   Causes of hypothermia

Environmental exposure
Immersion
Trauma
Shock
Sepsis
Iatrogenic causes (medical transport, treatment)
Alcohol and drugs (barbiturates, etc.)
Anorexia nervosa
Malnutrition (tropical hypothermia)
Hypoglycemia
Water intoxication
Burns and dermatoses
Hypothyroidism, hypoadrenalism
Hypothalamic lesions

With the exception of adolescents, children are less likely than adults to suffer hypothermia because of self-impairment (with alcohol or drugs) or mental illness. More often than adults, however, children suffer from cold during the process of rescue and medical resuscitation, transport and treatment. Severe cold is not required to produce significant hypothermia; any combination of cold, wet, wind, illness or injury can precipitate dangerous cooling.

MECHANISMS OF HEAT LOSS

Heat is lost from the human body by five basic mechanisms; an understanding of these is important to treatment as well as to prevention of hypothermia.

Radiation

The chief source of heat loss under most conditions is radiation of heat energy at the speed of light from the body's surface to surrounding objects. Under an open sky, heat actually radiates into outer space. Designed for heat regulation, human skin is a near-perfect radiator; its emissivity approaches the maximum value of 1.0. The spheroid shape of human head creates a highly effective source for heat loss, such that up to 75% of heat loss at $-15°C$ can occur through the head. Radiation of heat increases as the ambient temperature decreases.

Conduction

Conduction forms the major source of heat loss during immersion, as water possesses both a conductivity and a specific heat many times that of air. Hypothermia may develop in water as warm as 18°C after prolonged immersion. Conduction causes wet clothing to lose most of its insulating properties. A patient lying on cold ground or snow also loses heat by conduction.

Convection

Convection represents heat carried away by the movement of air next to the skin. In still conditions convection can account for up to 25% of lost body heat, and wind chill represents the very real increase in cooling caused by increased convection (for example, a 63 kph (35 mph) wind increases convective heat loss 14-fold).

Evaporation and respiration

Evaporation at rest (insensible loss) represents only a few per cent of the body's heat expenditure, but at its maximum can waste up to six times the amount of heat produced at the basal metabolic rate. Respiration causes heat loss by several of the above mechanisms, accounting for about 14% of heat loss at rest and much more with increases in exertion or in altitude, especially in cold, dry air.

PHYSIOLOGY

Decreased core temperature affects all body systems. The major changes in physiology and related symptoms are shown in Table 4.2. At body temperatures greater than approximately 32°C, compensatory mechanisms seek to restore normothermia. Below this temperature, compensatory mechanisms begin to fail, leading to loss of protective mechanisms, decreased thermogenesis and the inability to rewarm spontaneously. Over the narrow range between approximately 29 and 31°C, patients begin to develop organ systems failure that may lead to fatal complications unless treated. In this same range signs such as cyanosis and shivering may be replaced by erythema and muscle rigidity, making the recognition of hypothermia less obvious in more severe cases.

Physiologic features of the most clinical importance stem from decreases in mental, cardiac, respiratory, metabolic and vasomotor function, as well as decreases in cardiac stability and blood volume. These changes may make the patient appear lifeless, but only in these more advanced stages does hypothermia have the potential to protect against anoxia. Survivors of prolonged submersion usually have had core temperatures below 28–30°C.[4]

Individual patients vary in their response to a given body temperature; in general neurologic findings such as pupillary reactivity tend to decrease with severe hypothermia. Some patients will demonstrate clouded mentation even with mild hypothermia; others have been responsive to voice or pain even at 20–27°C.[5] Changes in mentation may lead to failure to retreat from a cold environment, and paradoxical undressing has been described. Apathetic,

Table 4.2 Physiology and clinical signs in hypothermia

Core temperature	Physiology	Signs
31–35°C	Increased BMR, VO$_2$ Vasoconstriction Tachycardia ADH increase	Shivering Cyanosis Clumsiness/dysarthria Diuresis
29–31°C	Decreasing BMR, VO$_2$ Decreased cerebral blood flow Acidosis or alkalosis Fluid shift Hypovolemia	Shivering stops Confusion/delirium Muscle rigidity Decreased or absent BP Decreased or absent pulse
25–29°C	Loss of thermoregulation Vasodilatation Decreased HR, SV, CO Slowed nerve conduction Suspended CNS activity Decreased cardiac conduction Increased cardiac irritability	Erythema/edema Stupor/coma Pulselessness Absent reflexes Fixed, dilated pupils Dysrhythmias Ventricular fibrillation
<25°C	Apnea Asystole	Appearance of death

BMR = Basal metabolic rate: VO$_2$ = oxygen consumption; ADH = antidiuretic hormone;
BP = blood pressure; HR = heart rate; SV = stroke volume; CO = cardiac output; CNS = central
nervous system. All changes shown may vary in temperature of onset. Not all signs
correspond to the physiologic changes shown on the same line of the table.

clumsy or combative behavior should signal leaders of youth outings to
suspect hypothermia.

Cardiac function declines with hypothermia, with decreases in stroke
volume, filling pressures, contractility, and heart rate. Cardiac changes also
vary from patient to patient. Although asystole and ventricular fibrillation
(VF) are common final rhythms in hypothermia, many patients have
demonstrated sinus rhythm, at least initially, despite severe hypothermia; one
patient had a heart rate of 50 beats/min and spontaneous respirations at
21.5°C.[6] On the electrocardiogram (ECG), a finding that is almost diagnostic
of hypothermia is the J-wave, or Osborn wave, appearing as a characteristic
hump at the J-point immediately after the QRS complex. This wave, although
nearly diagnostic of hypothermia, is not universal; it has only been seen in
somewhere between 11 and 80% of different series. Numerous other ECG
changes may occur.

Metabolic processes slow by approximately 6% for each decrease of 1°C in
body temperature; by 28°C the basal metabolic rate has fallen by approximately half. Decreases in ventilation may make breathing slow and shallow.
Oxygen delivery to tissues is further limited by decreased dissociation of
oxyhemoglobin due to cold. Of course, oxygen consumption also decreases;
protection against hypoxia results directly from slowed cellular metabolism.
Although this slowing of metabolism has been attributed to a 'diving reflex'
similar to that seen in sea mammals, some have found no evidence for such

a reflex in human beings. In any event an apparent requirement for survival would be that oxygen demand should decrease before hypoxia becomes critical. This means that rapid cooling with a preserved circulation carries a better prognosis than slow cooling after circulatory arrest.[7]

Renal effects of hypothermia combine to cause a marked cold diuresis, due both to a metabolic reduction in active tubular reabsorption and to decreased production of antidiuretic hormone. The latter results from peripheral vasoconstriction in early hypothermia which causes central volume receptors to perceive a volume excess. This apparent excess is augmented in cases of immersion by the hydrostatic pressure of the surrounding water.[8] The hypovolemia brought on by this diuresis is aggravated by a marked extravasation of intravascular fluid; the blood becomes thickened and sludges in small vessels, and vasodilation combines with the increasing rigidity of skeletal muscle to make palpation of pulses or measurement of blood pressure difficult in severely hypothermic patients even when circulation persists. Variable physiologic findings include hypo- or hyperglycemia, metabolic alkalosis or acidosis, and hypo- or hyperkalemia.

A crucial consequence of these changes in cardiovascular and metabolic function is that severely hypothermic patients may satisfy their metabolic demands even in the presence of marked hypoventilation, bradycardia, or hypotension. Because over-aggressive treatment of these findings has been linked at least anecdotally to cardiac arrest, these facts bear on resuscitation of severely hypothermic patients.

Several issues may pertain to sudden death after rescue. 'Afterdrop' is the well-known tendency of body temperature to decrease for a time even after a patient is removed from a cold environment. In part this may be due to the return of cold blood from the periphery to the core, which would suggest that peripheral rewarming and the resultant increase in peripheral circulation could increase afterdrop. On the other hand, work with solid models and with blood flow in volunteers suggests that conduction of heat from the core to the periphery would cause afterdrop even without the circulation of blood; that is, that afterdrop would occur regardless of method of warming. That both models possess some validity is borne out by the fact that afterdrop does indeed occur regardless of rewarming method, but may be decreased when peripheral warming is withheld.

Even more critical in death after rescue is 'rewarming shock'. The markedly collapsed circulation and depressed myocardium mentioned above will not be able to meet the increased demands occasioned by rewarming, increased peripheral vasodilation, renewed metabolism, and (in cases of immersion) the removal of the ambient hydrostatic pressure.[8] In addition, experts cite as causes of some cases of sudden death after rescue rough handling, excessive therapeutic manipulation, the administration of cold fluids, and exertion by the patient.

DIAGNOSIS

Only two items are required to diagnose hypothermia: a low-recording thermometer and a high index of suspicion. Standard clinical thermometers do not record below 34°C, that is, they will not reveal any genuine cases of hypothermia. Although low-recording thermometers should be stocked routinely by accident departments and others seeing patients exposed to cold, alternatives may be useful as well. These include temperature probes such as those used in newborn nurseries or departments of anesthesiology, and even ordinary glass laboratory or room thermometers. Reference core temperatures are measured by direct tympanic thermometry; the use of indirect reflectance tympanic thermometers has been shown to reflect core temperature at least in some studies.[9] Esophageal probes reflect mediastinal (cardiac) temperatures, and may be more easily placed than bladder probes. Rectal temperatures, though subject to artifacts and time delays in reflecting central temperature, are adequate if measured deep (at least 10 cm) in the rectal vault. Oral, axillary, and cutaneous temperatures are unreliable in the hypothermic patient.

Hypothermia is not usually missed in the shivering patient just pulled from a snowbank, but can easily be overlooked if the symptoms are more insidious (as in colder patients) or if the cold insult is less obvious. Any child exposed to any combination of severe injury or illness, or to wind or wet or cold, is at risk for hypothermia.

Hypothermia is categorized both by degree (Table 4.1) and by the rapidity of onset. *Acute* hypothermia develops over minutes, as in cases of icy-water immersion. *Submersion* hypothermia adds the injuries associated with near-drowning to acute hypothermia. *Subacute* hypothermia develops over a few hours or more, often as a result of exposure outdoors. *Chronic* hypothermia develops over days of exposure to milder temperatures; except in young infants this form is less common in children.

COMPLICATIONS

Hypothermia can give rise to various complications, some of which are listed in Table 4.3. Those complications that are especially common (pulmonary disease, central nervous system dysfunction, coagulopathy, and renal failure for instance) are also likely to mandate intensive care even if resuscitation is successful. This is especially true if other injuries are present due to trauma, a frequent precipitant of hypothermia, or to near-drowning. The treatment of these complications is little different in the survivor of hypothermia than in other patients, and needs no elaboration here other than to emphasize that the oft-noted tendency of hypothermia survivors to show only gradual neurologic recovery[2,4] would indicate that maximal reasonable care be provided and that physicians not be too quick to offer a neurologic prognosis in such cases.

Table 4.3 Possible complications of hypothermia

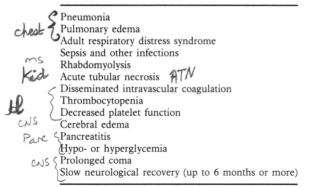

chest { Pneumonia
       Pulmonary edema
       Adult respiratory distress syndrome
       Sepsis and other infections
ms   Rhabdomyolysis
Kid   Acute tubular necrosis ATN
       Disseminated intravascular coagulation
       Thrombocytopenia
       Decreased platelet function
CNS   Cerebral edema
Panc   Pancreatitis
       Hypo- or hyperglycemia
CNS   Prolonged coma
       Slow neurological recovery (up to 6 months or more)

TREATMENT

The paradox of hypothermia is especially acute in treatment: only the severely hypothermic patient, who is most difficult to treat and may appear beyond treatment, will have the potential to benefit from the hypoxic protection that hypothermia sometimes confers. Standard clinical systems for predicting outcome, such as the Glasgow Coma Scale, fail in the presence of severe hypothermia. A 2-year-old girl survived intact after more than an hour's submersion in icy water.[2] A Swiss climber underwent at least 3 h of asystole at 19°C, including 1 hour without cardiopulmonary resuscitation (CPR), yet was able to return to work 2 weeks later.[10] Patients have survived temperatures as low as 9°C in induced hypothermia and 15°C in accidental hypothermia.

Treatment during rescue involves recognition of hypothermia and prevention of further heat loss. In remote locations, gentle handling plus provision of shelter, dry insulation, and some form of external rewarming may be all that can be achieved. Medical transport introduces new challenges. Rewarming during prehospital treatment has been criticized because it precedes the availability of sophisticated patient support measures. External rewarming can indeed be harmful in severe hypothermia. Safer rewarming methods available in prehospital care, such as heated humidified oxygen, have only limited ability to transfer heat.[11] Yet undue emphasis on avoiding rewarming during transport may explain in part why patients tend to arrive colder at the hospital than when they left the scene. Reasonable measures to prevent further heat loss during transport include heating of transport vehicles, removal of cold or wet clothing, provision of dry blankets, warming of intravenous fluids, and provision of heated humidified oxygen. Gentle handling is again important.

Because of the physiologic changes described above, indications for life support measures may be altered in severe hypothermia. When a patient is known to be severely hypothermic, most authors feel that any spontaneous breathing is probably adequate, even if shallow or slow. If no breathing is present after a careful assessment, an airway and breathing should be provided, using bag-mask ventilation and then, if necessary, an endotracheal tube. Muscle rigidity may make these measures more difficult. Although intubation has been associated with VF in isolated cases, experience in animals[12] and in large series of human cases[3] suggests that intubation is safe in hypothermic patients. Overventilation should probably be avoided.

Indications for CPR are more problematic. Because even a bradycardic, hypotensive circulation may satisfy the reduced metabolic demands of hypothermia; because CPR has been associated with the onset of VF; because preservation of a circulating rhythm eases rewarming;[6] and because CPR is even less effective at providing circulation during hypothermia,[13] almost all experts agree that CPR should be withheld in the severely hypothermic patient with a pulse, regardless of heart rate or blood pressure.

A randomized, controlled trial of CPR in severe hypothermia would be difficult. Recent recommendations reflect a consensus among experts.[14–17] If core temperature is unknown, CPR must be started for apparent cardiac arrest, although extra care may be used in efforts to detect a pulse in cases of suspected hypothermia. If any pulse is present when the core temperature is known to be below 30°C, CPR can be withheld (or stopped if it was previously begun for apparent bradycardia or hypotension). Some authors would also withhold CPR at these temperatures if an ECG monitor shows presence of a narrow-complex perfusing rhythm, even in the absence of a palpable pulse.[15]

The desire to withhold CPR in severe hypothermia must be tempered by the fact that evidence that CPR precipitates VF is largely circumstantial, that accurate temperature assessment is not often practicable when the decision to begin CPR needs to be made, and that CPR in hypothermia may not lose its effectiveness over time as it does in normothermia.[13] Until more is known about the mechanisms of CPR in hypothermia, standard rates and techniques should be employed.

The requirement for volume expansion will be obvious in view of the hypovolemia and rewarming shock discussed above, and has proven clinically important.[18] Fluids at room temperature are not thermally neutral, but rather are colder than all but the coldest patients. Administration of such fluids further cools the patient and may precipitate VF. Isotonic solutions (0.9% sodium chloride or lactated Ringer solution) should be warmed to approximately 40°C and infused rapidly in boluses of 20 ml/kg as required. Central venous pressure monitoring can aid in estimating the adequacy of volume restoration. Pneumatic antishock garments may be ineffective or, theoretically, harmful in hypothermia.

Medications may demonstrate no effect, or altered effects, in the cold patient, yet persist in the body due to suppressed metabolism and elimination, becoming active only after rewarming when their effects will no longer be desirable.[17] Glucose should be administered as soon as possible, because hypoglycemia can be a frequent concomitant of hypothermia. Drugs of possible usefulness include the vasopressors, especially dopamine, which have been shown to have some effect during hypothermia.[19,20] Lignocaine appears safe, if of unclear efficacy. Bretylium tosylate has been associated with some reports of spontaneous defibrillation;[21] on the other hand this effect could not be demonstrated in animals,[22] nor could a protective effect against the onset of VF.[23] The fact that some animal subjects developed VF during infusion of bretylium weighs against too-ready use for prophylaxis of VF, but use in patients already fibrillating may prove beneficial. Drugs not generally recommended include sodium bicarbonate,[24] corticosteroids, 'prophylactic' antibiotics, and insulin (hyperglycemia, unlike hypoglycemia, resolves spontaneously with rewarming).

Electrical defibrillation often proves unsuccessful in severe hypothermia. After three initial attempts, it may be best to withhold further shocks until body temperature rises above 30°C[14] as electrical defibrillation is more likely to succeed above this temperature, and spontaneous defibrillation may obviate the need for repeated unsuccessful defibrillation.

The hypothermic patient should have repeated or continuous monitoring of the core temperature, ECG tracing, and vital signs including blood pressure; serum glucose, amylase, and electrolyte values; arterial blood gases, urinalysis and urine output; as well as ethanol, thyroid hormone, and toxin screens when indicated and appropriate efforts to define possible infection. Arterial blood gas measurements had in the past been corrected for body temperature; blood gas machines test samples at 37°C, so tables were constructed to show the 'actual' gas tensions and pH at the patient's temperature. Correction for hypothermia produces a higher pH and lower carbon dioxide and oxygen tensions. Beyond its intuitive logic, arguments have been put forward to support temperature correction.[11] Recent analysis of clinical, physiochemical, and even comparative physiologic data suggests, however, that uncorrected pH and carbon dioxide measurements better represent the altered chemistry of cold systems, allow for easier diagnosis and analysis of derangements, and provide better outcomes. These complex arguments are summarized by Delaney and coauthors,[25] who point out the consequences of correction or non-correction and demonstrate the advantages of the former. Correction of oxygen tensions for hypothermia may not be harmful, but will seldom alter the recommendation to administer maximal oxygen concentrations to children during resuscitation. Pulse oximetry and transcutaneous measurement of gas tensions are inaccurate in the presence of decreased perfusion.

REWARMING

The question of how to rewarm hypothermic patients had for a long time remained controversial; much of the debate centered on the rate of rewarming, with different recommendations arising from studies of different populations. In part this controversy stemmed from the simple fact that no single method or rate of rewarming can be applied with equal efficacy and safety to an elderly pensioner rescued from an unheated flat, an inebriated adolescent found sleeping in the snow, and a young child pulled from an icy pond. Even using the same techniques within one class of hypothermic patients, rewarming rates can vary widely. If nothing else, the patient with an intact circulation will rewarm more quickly than the patient with circulatory arrest. A sensible note is sounded by Myers and co-workers, who write: 'Mortality rates, rather than rewarming rates, should dictate the choice of therapy'.[11]

Rewarming methods are divided into three general classes, outlined in Table 4.4. Passive rewarming, the provision of insulation in a warm room, requires that patients have spontaneous thermogenesis and be quite stable; it has proven most useful in the elderly victim of mild, chronic hypothermia. Not surprisingly, passive rewarming has been found to carry a high mortality rate in adult victims of severe hypothermia,[26] and in neonatal hypothermia, active rewarming produces better results.[27]

Active rewarming (also called surface rewarming) had initially been supported by reports of the infamous Nazi experiments on hypothermia, now seen to be wholly invalid.[28] These methods do provide some advantages, including relative rapidity, easy availability, and technical simplicity. Early reports of severe hazards[29] are now attributed in part to insufficient awareness of the need for supportive care and volume resuscitation.[30] The techniques also carry disadvantages; surface warming (with hot packs warmer than 45°C) has burned some patients, partly due to decreased cutaneous perfusion. The same decrease in cutaneous perfusion slows transfer of the heat to the body's core. Heating blankets and especially hot baths decrease access to the patient. Most importantly, external rewarming increases metabolic rates before the circulation is prepared to support them, and produces peripheral

Table 4.4   Rewarming methods

Passive	Active external	Core
Warm room (21–23°C)	Warmed blankets	Warm intravenous fluids (36–40°C)
Dry blankets	Chemical hot packs	Warmed airway mist (40°C)
Monitor	Plumbed blankets/pads	Warmed lavage (40°C)
	Radiant warmers/lights	Gastric/colonic
	Hot baths/immersion*	Esophageal/bladder
		Peritoneal dialysis†
		Hemodialysis
		Closed pleural lavage
		Extracorporeal blood warming
		Extravascular shunts
		Heart–lung pump

Core methods are listed approximately in order of increasing efficacy.
*Immersion of just the trunk has been suggested to decrease afterdrop.
†Peritoneal dialysis may be performed using aliquots of 50 ml/kg of a 1.5% dialysis solution warmed to 40°C with quick dwell times.

vasodilation, returning cold, acidotic blood to the central circulation and potentiating afterdrop, rewarming shock, and VF. Despite these concerns, external techniques work well to rewarm many patients with mild hypothermia, and to prevent cooling during medical treatment. External rewarming may be the only method readily available in remote locations or in small health facilities. Even in patients with more severe hypothermia but preserved circulation, effective use of external rewarming continues to be reported where no other methods are available.

Core rewarming prevents or decreases many of the problems associated with external rewarming; furthermore, some methods are simple, and most provide patient support. Core rewarming is especially important for the patient in severe hypothermia or the patient in circulatory arrest. The simplest core rewarming techniques, heating of intravenous fluids and humidified oxygen, transfer little net heat to the patient,[11] but do prevent further cooling and provide patient support. Warming of intravenous solutions is not as simple as it sounds. Solutions in plastic bags can be warmed in a microwave oven or stored in warm cabinets; even when warmed solutions are used, one must employ short lengths of intravenous tubing and high flow rates to prevent cooling before the fluid enters the patient.[31] Only a few commercial blood warmers provide adequate heating of fluids, and many limit rates of flow.[32] Warmed intravenous solutions and heated, humidified oxygen, while necessary, will be sufficient by themselves to rewarm only fairly mild cases of hypothermia or those with preserved circulation and thermogenesis.

More substantial transfer of heat occurs when greater volumes of warm fluid contact larger body surfaces. Warmed gastric (or colonic) lavage is a technique accessible to most health facilities. Esophageal warming devices have been used with success.[33] Warm peritoneal dialysis can be used in many hospitals.[34] Warm hemodialysis can be helpful especially when an overdose of drugs (e.g. barbiturates) is involved. More recently, continuous closed pleural lavage using two left-sided thoracostomy tubes has been reported to produce more rapid rates of rewarming.[35,36] Use of high-flow fluid warmers appears to be the easiest way to supply the large volumes of heated saline needed in this technique. The relative simplicity of this method may recommend it to most practitioners as an alternative to open thoracostomy and mediastinal irrigation, although the latter technique has been used successfully. Many case reports now document the successful use of extracorporeal blood rewarming, using either the standard heart–lung machine employed in cardiac surgery[2] or, in those with intact circulation, newer arteriovenous or venovenous rewarming devices.[37,38] These newer methods may bring the advantages of extracorporeal rewarming to patients with milder degrees of hypothermia, at least in intensive-care settings. For those patients with severe or profound hypothermia and little or no circulation of blood, the use of the heart–lung pump offers the advantages of extremely rapid core rewarming while additionally restoring the circulation, providing oxygenation, reversing hypovolemia and hemoconcentration, and decreasing stress on the myocardium. These advantages have made extracorporeal circulation the treatment of choice in hypothermic arrest.[39] Even where a centre with a pediatric heart–lung team is some distance away, it should be borne in mind that such rewarming has revived patients even after 3 h of transport.[10] The alternative in cases of hypothermic arrest is often hours of fruitless rewarming, all the while performing ineffective CPR.

Although extracorporeal rewarming can be remarkably effective, it is not a panacea. The publication mainly of successful case reports gives an unrealistic picture of the odds of success. Effective rewarming will not revive patients who are dead,[40] nor will it protect the patient against lethal injuries or complications of the original illness or injury. Where safer and less invasive methods suffice to rewarm a patient, extracorporeal circulation can be avoided; furthermore the unavailability of this technique should not dissuade the practitioner from aggressive attempts at rewarming using other methods, which continue to produce successful outcomes even in some cases of profound hypothermia. The choice of rewarming methods should be individualized to each patient. Patients with severe or profound hypothermia require core rewarming; when rapid rewarming is appropriate, which includes most pediatric cases, methods should be selected which can transfer large amounts of heat to the patient. Moderate hypothermia with an intact circulation may respond to heated intravenous fluids and heated, humidified oxygen plus gentle external rewarming. Mild hypothermia will usually respond to external measures alone. For any patient, if the methods chosen do not produce rewarming, more aggressive techniques should be selected.

Are there patients in whom rewarming attempts can be assumed to be futile in advance? With reports of intact survival after cold submersion for 66 min,[2] or of survival after 6.5 h of CPR,[40] it is clear that any patient with a chance of hypothermic protection deserves an attempt at rewarming. On the other hand, hypothermia does not protect against lethal injuries other than hypoxia, and patients who are genuinely dead are often found hypothermic. Attempts are now underway to identify chemical markers of death such as extreme hyperkalemia or hyperammonemia;[40] although promising, these methods cannot be regarded as absolute until confirmatory work shows a clear boundary between living and dead patients. Failure to restore a perfusing rhythm within approximately 30 min of rewarming to 32°–35° C makes further efforts unlikely to be rewarding.

In near-drowning, it is also clear now that only the coldest water affords patients a chance of hypothermic protection. Orlowski[42] has noted that all reported cases of survival after more than 15 min submersion occurred in water colder than 10°C, and that 16 of 17 cases probably involved water temperatures less than 5°C. This observation suggests that the term 'ice-water drowning' replace 'cold-water drowning' in discussions of possible hypothermic protection. Even in ice-water drowning, patients may succumb to hypoxia as well as lung injury, multisystem failure, or traumatic complications.

PREVENTION

Knowing that hypothermic protection against anoxia is uncommon, that hypothermia itself is dangerous, and that treatment is difficult and by no means certain to succeed, it is clear that the best measure to combat hypothermia is prevention. Two major causes of accidental hypothermia in children, trauma and drowning accidents, have been the focus of extensive preventive campaigns in pediatrics; those concerned with the welfare of children must continue to work through legislative and educational channels to reduce the toll of death and disability from these accidents. Standard teachings in 'drown-proofing' may have the head held in the water, or the body extended, or both. Other water safety programs emphasize strong swimming skills. Neither approach is effective in icy water, where heat loss is the major enemy and swimming skills are rapidly rendered useless by incoordination or involuntary thrashing brought on by cold. Those exposed to cold water should be taught the heat-escape-lessening position (HELP) with the arms folded tightly to the anterior axillary line and the knees flexed to the chest. The maintenance of this position requires the use of a flotation device, or life vest; this is important in cold water even for the strongest swimmers, not only to allow flotation in the proper position but also to decrease heat loss through the trunk.

Those interested in youth sports and outdoor activities or in public safety must increase the public's awareness of the risks of hypothermia. Special clothing and equipment designed to prevent hypothermia will only be useful to young people if it is available to them and they are instructed in its use. For those in rescue services and ambulance companies, recognition and prevention of hypothermia are of special importance. Within clinics, accident departments, and hospitals, the development of hypothermia during resuscitation must be seen as a serious but preventable iatrogenic complication.

KEY POINTS FOR CLINICAL PRACTICE

- The obvious physical findings of hypothermia disappear in severe cases, leading to missed diagnoses.
- Patients with core temperatures below approximately 30°C may have a chance of protection against hypoxia, but also lose their compensatory mechansims and fall prey to potentially fatal complications of hypothermia.
- Core rewarming techniques are preferred for victims of severe hypothermia; methods providing a large heat transfer, such as closed pleural lavage, are more rapidly effective.
- Hypothermic patients in cardiac arrest are most easily rewarmed using extracorporeal circulation.

REFERENCES

1 Siebke H, Breivik H, Rød T, Lind B. Survival after 40 minutes' submersion without

cerebral sequelae. Lancet 1975; 1: 1275–1277

2 Bolte RG, Black PG, Bowers RS, Thorne JK, Corneli HM. The use of extracorporeal rewarming in a child submerged for 66 minutes. JAMA 1988; 260: 377–379

3 Danzl DF, Pozos RS, Auerbach PS, Glazer S, Goetz W, Johnson E. Multicenter hypothermia survey. Ann Emerg Med 1987; 16: 1042–1055

4 Young R, Zalneraitis EL, Dooling EC. Neurological outcome in cold water drowning. JAMA 1980; 244: 1233–1235

5 O'Keeffe KM. Accidental hypothermia: a review of 62 cases. JACEP (J Am Coll Emerg Phys) 1977; 6: 491–496

6 Kugelberg J, Schüller H, Berg B, Kallum B. Treatment of accidental hypothermia. Scand J Thorac Cardiovasc Surg 1967; 1: 142–146

7 Orlowski JP. Drowning, near-drowning, and ice-water submersions. Pediatr Clin North Am 1987; 34: 75–92

8 Golden FS. Problems of immersion. Br J Hosp Med 1980; 24: 371–374

9 Jakobbson J, Nilsson A, Carlsson L. Core temperature measured in the auricular canal: comparison between four different tympanic thermometers. Acta Anaesthesiol Scand 1992; 36: 819–834

10 Althaus U, Aeberhard P, Schüpbach P, Nachbur BH, Mühlemann W. Management of profound accidental hypothermia with cardiorespiratory arrest. Ann Surg 1982; 195: 492–495

11 Myers RA, Britten JS, Cowley RA. Hypothermia: quantitative aspects of therapy. JACEP (J Am Coll Emerg Phys) 1979; 8: 523–527

12 Gillen JP, Vogel MF, Holterman RK, Skiendzielewski JJ. Ventricular fibrillation during orotracheal intubation of hypothermic dogs. Ann Emerg Med 1986; 15: 412–416

13 Maningas PA, DeGuzman LR, Hollenbach SJ, Volk KA, Bellamy RF. Regional blood flow during hypothermic arrest. Ann Emerg Med 1986; 15: 390–396

14 Emergency Cardiac Care Committee and Subcommittees, American Heart Association. Special resuscitation situations. JAMA 1992; 268: 2242–2250

15 Robinson M, Seward PN. Environmental hypothermia in children. Pediatr Emerg Care 1986; 2: 254–257

16 Steinman AM. Cardiopulmonary resuscitation and hypothermia. Circulation 1986; 74: IV29–32

17 Ornato JP. Special resuscitation situations; near drowning, traumatic injury, electric shock, and hypothermia. Circulation 1986; 74: IV23–26

18 Ledingham IM, Mone JG. Treatment of accidental hypothermia: a prospective clinical study. Br Med J 1980; 280: 1102–1105

19 Nicodemus HF, Chaney RD, Herold R. Hemodynamic effects of inotropes during hypothermia and rapid rewarming. Crit Care Med 1981; 9: 325–328

20 Riishede L, Nielsen KF. Myocardial effects of adrenaline, isoprenaline and dobutamine at hypothermic conditions. Pharmacol Toxicol 1990; 66: 354–360

21 Danzl DF, Sowers MB, Vicario SJ, Thomas DM, Miller JW. Chemical ventricular defibrillation in severe accidental hypothermia. Ann Emerg Med 1982; 11: 698–699

22 Elenbaas RM, Mattson K, Cole H, Steele M, Ryan J, Robinson W. Bretylium in hypothermia-induced ventricular fibrillation in dogs. Ann Emerg Med 1984; 13: 994–999

23 Murphy K, Nowak RM, Tomlanovich MC. Use of bretylium tosylate as prophylaxis and treatment in hypothermic ventricular fibrillation in the canine model. Ann Emerg Med 1986; 15: 1160–1166

24 Swain JA. Hypothermia and blood pH. A review. Arch Intern Med 1988; 148: 1643–1646

25 Delaney KA, Howland MA, Vassallo S, Goldfrank LR. Assessment of acid–base disturbances in hypothermia and their physiologic consequences. Ann Emerg Med 1989; 18: 72–82

26 White JD. Hypothermia: the Bellevue experience. Ann Emerg Med 1982; 11: 417–424

27 Kaplan M, Eidelman AI. Improved prognosis in severely hypothermic newborn infants treated by rapid rewarming. J Pediatr 1984; 105: 470–474

28 Berger RL. Nazi science—the Dachau hypothermia experiments. N Engl J Med 1990; 322: 1435–1440

29 Duguid H, Simpson RG, Stowers JM. Accidental hypothermia. Lancet 1961; 2: 1213–1219

30 Lloyd EL. Hypothermia: the cause of death after rescue. Alaska Med 1984; 26: 74–76

31 Faries G, Johnston C, Pruitt KM, Plouff RT. Temperature relationship to distance and flow rate of warmed I.V. fluids. Ann Emerg Med 1991; 20: 1198–1200

32 Flancbaum L, Trooskin SZ, Pedersen H. Evaluation of blood-warming devices with the apparent thermal clearance. Ann Emerg Med 1989; 18: 355–359

33 Kristensen G, Drenck NE, Jordening H. Simple system for central rewarming of hypothermic patients. Lancet 1986; 2: 8521–8522

34 Jessen K, Hagelsten JO. Peritoneal dialysis in the treatment of profound accidental hypothermia. Aviat Space Environ Med 1978; 49: 426–429

35 Hall KN, Syverud SA. Closed thoracic cavity lavage in the treatment of severe hypothermia in human beings. Ann Emerg Med 1990; 19: 204–206

36 Iversen RJ, Atkin SH, Jaker MA, Quadrel MA, Tortella BJ, Odom JW. Successful CPR in a severely hypothermic patient using continuous thoracostomy lavage. Ann Emerg Med 1990; 19: 1335–1337

37 Gregory JS, Bergstein JM, Aprahamian C, Wittmann DH, Quebbeman EJ. Comparison of three methods of rewarming from hypothermia: advantages of extracorporeal blood warming. J Trauma 1991; 31: 1247–1251

38 Gentilello LM, Cobean RA, Offner PJ, Soderberg RW, Jurkovich GJ. Continuous arteriovenous rewarming: rapid reversal of hypothermia in critically ill patients. J Trauma 1992; 32: 316–325

39 Keatinge WR. Hypothermia: dead or alive? Br Med J 1991; 302: 3–4

40 Hauty MG, Esrig BC, Hill JG, Long WB. Prognostic factors in severe accidental hypothermia: experience from the Mt. Hood tragedy. J Trauma 1987; 27: 1107–1112

41 Lexow K. Severe accidental hypothermia; survival after 6 hours 30 minutes of cardiopulmonary resuscitation. Arctic Med Res 1991; 6: 112–11

42 Orlowski JP. Drowning, near-drowning, and ice-water drowning. JAMA 1988; 260: 390–391

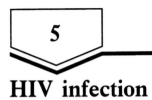

HIV infection

M.-L. Newell   D. M. Gibb

GLOBAL IMPACT OF AIDS

Over the last 12 years, the acquired immunodeficiency syndrome (AIDS) epidemic has emerged as a disease with social, political, medical and economic implications. By the year 2000, as many as 40 million people may be infected with human immunodeficiency virus (HIV).[1] Although more than 90% of these will live in sub-Saharan Africa, South and South-East Asia, Latin America, and the Caribbean, increasing numbers of cases are being reported from most countries, including the USA and Europe.[2] By the end of the decade there could be at least 10 million HIV-infected children. In addition, during the 1990s, mothers or both parents of more than 10 million children will have died from HIV infection.[3] In some parts of Africa, the effects of paediatric HIV infection have already negated the gains made in child survival due to the expanded programmes of immunization and oral rehydration schemes.

In Africa, where most infected people have acquired HIV heterosexually, approximately equal numbers of men and women are infected. However, this situation may be changing and a recent review of three population studies showed that the infection rate was considerably higher in women than in men.[4] In the USA and Europe heterosexual transmission is increasing and the male-to-female ratio of reported AIDS cases in adults has decreased from 7 in 1989 to 6 in 1992. As mother-to-child transmission is the major route of acquisition of HIV infection for children, the rise in heterosexual transmission is likely to result in a parallel increase in the number of children with HIV infection.

By September 1992, 11 182 adult women and 3577 children from 31 European countries had been diagnosed with AIDS.[2] More than 50% of women acquired the infection through intravenous drug use, although 30% had become infected through heterosexual contact; the majority are of child-bearing age. Most children with AIDS were reported from France (411), Italy (322) and Spain (434). Eighty-nine children with AIDS have been reported from the UK. The 1948 children reported from Romania were uniquely infected through contaminated blood and syringes, and highlight the need for continued vigilance in the use of blood and blood products.

As the incubation time of AIDS can be long, knowledge of the prevalence of HIV infection provides more relevant information. Thus, unlinked anonymous testing of blood taken for other purposes has provided the most useful information in the monitoring of the epidemic. Such studies are now in progress in the USA and many parts of Europe using bloods collected from women antenatally, from neonates (which reflects the prevalence of infection in their mothers), in genitourinary medicine clinics or in casualty. The former two are particularly relevant for children as vertical transmission from mother to child is the main mode of acquisition of infection in children.

Further information about the extent of the problem comes from registers where HIV-seropositive children are reported by clinicians.[5-7] In the UK, linkage of confidential obstetrical and paediatric registers with results from the unlinked, anonymous neonatal screening programme provides a unique opportunity to evaluate the extent of coverage of the registries.[8]

In the British Isles, 527 children born to HIV-infected mothers have been reported, of whom 189 have definitive HIV infection. The majority of infected children were reported from London, although comparison of the register with the results of anonymous neonatal tests indicates that only 17% of infected pregnant women are recognized by the clinicians.

PREGNANCY AND HIV INFECTION

To date, there is no evidence that pregnancy has an adverse effect on the progression of HIV disease in asymptomatic women,[9] but further research is needed, especially for women with HIV-related manifestations.

Whereas in Europe and the USA prospective studies[10] have not demonstrated adverse effects of maternal HIV infection on the fetus and newborn (abortions, low birth weight), low birth weight has been reported in a higher proportion of babies born to HIV-infected women compared to those born to HIV-negative controls in both Africa and Haiti.[10] This finding could reflect the poor social and health status of HIV-infected mothers from these regions, rather than being due to a direct effect of HIV infection on the fetus.

There are advantages for both mother and baby if the woman's HIV status is known during pregnancy. She may wish to terminate the pregnancy, although there is some evidence to suggest that knowledge of HIV infection status does not affect a woman's decision regarding termination of pregnancy. When a woman chooses to continue the pregnancy close collaboration between paediatric and obstetric staff is important so that accurate information can be given about the risk of transmitting HIV to her child, and advice about breast-feeding and follow-up of her child. Ideally, the paediatrician should be involved before the delivery so that a good relationship can be formed with the mother before the child is born.

VERTICAL TRANSMISSION

Vertical transmission rates

The calculation of the rate of vertical transmission must be based on a cohort of children known to be born to an HIV-infected mother, followed prospectively from birth, to avoid bias towards those with symptoms.[10] Therefore, vertical transmission rates cannot be calculated from registries. Estimates of the rate of vertical transmission of HIV infection from mother to child, from published papers of prospective studies, range from 7 to 39%. In Europe the rate of mother-to-child transmisson is 15–20%.[7,8,10,11] The vertical transmission rates from mother to child reported from Africa appear to be higher, and are in the order of 30%.[10]

Timing of acquisition

Transmission of HIV infection can occur before, during or after birth; however, the relative importance of each of these routes is unknown.[10] Intrauterine infection is suggested by the identification of virus from fetal tissue, placenta and cord blood. In addition, the very early onset of AIDS in some infants suggests intrauterine acquisition of infection. The increased exchange of blood between mother and child at the time of delivery, as well as the presence of virus in cervical secretions may result in transmission during delivery. Transmission of HIV through breast milk has been described in situations where the mother acquired the infection shortly after birth, following a contaminated blood transfusion or through heterosexual contact. The additional risk of transmission of HIV through breast milk from a mother who was already antibody-positive during pregnancy is less, but still substantial.

Maternal characteristics and vertical transmission

Recent information confirms previous circumstantial evidence that maternal characteristics may influence vertical transmission rates[10,12] (Table 5.1). In the European Collaborative Study vertical transmission was associated with AIDS in the mother but not with less advanced HIV-related manifestations.[11] The rate of transmission increased sharply when the CD4 count dropped below $700/mm^3$ or the CD4:CD8 ratio below 0.6, and was strongly associated with p24-antigenaemia. These findings suggest that maternal clinical and immunological status during pregnancy and the duration of her infection influence the viral load and infectivity, thereby affecting vertical transmission. This is also suggested by the results of a study in Kinshasa, Zaire where infants born to mothers with low CD4 counts were more likely to be infected than infants born to women with CD4 counts above $400/mm^3$.[10] In Sweden mothers of infected children had been infected for longer and were more

Table 5.1   Possible risk factors for mother-to-child transmission

---

Viral characteristics
Background infections, sexually transmitted diseases
Genetic
Primary infection during pregnancy
Advanced HIV disease
Immunological status
Premature delivery
Mode of delivery
Breast-feeding

HIV = Human immunodeficiency virus.

likely to be symptomatic and/or to have low CD4 cell counts at follow-up than mothers of uninfected children.[10] However, in a study in the USA no association was reported between transmission and pre-delivery levels of maternal CD4 cells, anti-p24 levels or neutralizing antibodies.[90] Other factors influencing viral load, such as primary infection, or factors stimulating the immune system such as other chronic infections, could also be important. It has been suggested that the presence of certain antibodies such as gp120 could protect the child against transmission of HIV.[10] However, these results have been refuted, and further studies are required.

Vertical transmission does not appear to be significantly associated with mode of acquisition of HIV infection, parity, race or age of mother at time of delivery, suggesting that these latter variables are not indicative of length of infection. [7,10,11]

Delivery and vertical transmission

In the European Collaborative Study most children were delivered vaginally, and the vertical transmission rate in this group was similar to that of children delivered by elective caesarean section.[11] It has been suggested that an elective caesarean delivery may reduce the rate of transmission because of a reduced exposure to contaminated blood or cervical secretions. However, published reports from prospective studies have not been able to confirm this and no significant difference in the vertical transmission rate according to mode of delivery has been reported.[10,11] There would be no justification from the data available to recommend elective caesarean section.

Prematurity has been associated with an increased risk of infection in the infant,[11] although this was not the case for children enrolled in the Italian register.[12] In the European Collaborative Study children born before 34 weeks' gestation were more likely to be infected than children born after longer gestation. The birth weight of these very premature infants was appropriate for gestational age, adjusted for maternal injecting drug use. The high frequency of HIV infection in children born before 34 weeks' gestation could be explained by the hypothesis that infants born before 34 weeks are more susceptible to intrapartum HIV-1 infection because of lower immunocompetence, and, possibly, lower levels of passively acquired antibodies. Alternatively it may be that in utero HIV infection causes premature delivery or that infectious women are more likely to transmit and to deliver prematurely or that concurrent infections may increase both the likelihood of infection and the risk of transmission. These latter hypotheses do not easily explain the sudden decrease in transmission rate after 34 weeks' gestation.

Breast-feeding and transmission of HIV

Transmission of HIV through breast milk has been described in situations where the mother acquired the infection shortly after birth, either through contaminated blood or through heterosexual contact. Mothers who seroconvert after the delivery have a high risk of transmitting HIV to their infants through breast-feeding, particularly if seroconversion occurs in the first 3 months after delivery. In the acute phase of primary infection, these women have a high virus load. It has been estimated that the risk of transmission of infection through breast-feeding in women infected postnatally is about 29% (95% confidence interval 16–42%).[14]

Recent evidence suggests that breast-feeding is also an important additional route of transmission in women already HIV-infected during or before pregnancy. It has been estimated that where the mother was infected prenatally the additional risk of transmission through breast-feeding, over and above transmission in utero or during delivery, is 14% (95% confidence interval 7–22%),[14] indicating that in Europe breast-feeding approximately doubles (from 14 to 28%) the risk of transmission from mother to child.

Early diagnosis

Whereas in adults and older children the diagnosis of HIV infection can reliably be made on the basis of detection of HIV antibodies, in children born to HIV-positive mothers the presence of passively acquired maternal antibodies, which cross the placenta and may be detected in the child up to 18 months after birth, makes the diagnosis of infection difficult. Thus, it is not until after this age that a positive HIV antibody test indicates definitive HIV infection in the child (Table 5.2).

HIV infection in the young infant can be diagnosed by the detection of virus or viral antigen from lymphocytes or free viral antigen in serum.[15] However, these tests are expensive, can only be done in specialized laboratories and are not widely available for routine diagnostic purposes. Also, not all cells will carry the virus and free antigen may not be present in an infected child. A failure to detect virus or antigen in a young, antibody-positive child does not exclude infection, but a positive virus or antigen test is likely to indicate infection.[16] It has recently been suggested that acid

Table 5.2 Diagnosis of HIV infection
in infants

Definitive
   Persistent HIV antibody after 18 months
   Development of AIDS
   p24 antigen or virus culture positive
Early diagnosis facilitated by:
   Viral tests
   Immunological tests
   Clinical manifestations

HIV = Human immunodeficiency virus,
AIDS = acquired immunodeficiency
     syndrome.

dissociation of p24 antigen–antibody complexes may make antigen tests more sensitive as a method of early diagnosis.[17] The introduction of the polymerase chain reaction (PCR) method of diagnosis of HIV infection, which amplifies viral genetic material, thus facilitating the detection of minute quantities of virus, will lead to an earlier diagnosis of infection. However, at the present time this remains a research tool, and further evaluation and standardization of the method are required. The detection of HIV-specific immunoglobulin A antibodies has been described as sensitive and specific at about 6 months of age.[15] The in vitro antibody production test in which the child's lymphocytes are separated and stimulated to produce their own HIV antibody can be useful after 2 months of age.[15]

Without a definitive virological diagnosis, the regular monitoring of immunoglobulins, CD4:CD8 ratio and clinical signs provides useful information to establish the HIV infection status in the child.[18] In order to make an early diagnosis, virological and immunological tests together with clinical examination should be performed in the neonatal period, at 6 weeks, 3 months, and thereafter at 3-monthly intervals. It should be noted that, even in the best laboratories, the sensitivity of viral tests for HIV is often less than 50% in the first week of life.[15] In experienced laboratories PCR and viral culture techniques are highly sensitive after 2–3 months of age.

If a viral test is positive, it should always be confirmed on a separate sample before information is given to the mother. Repeatedly negative tests in an immunologically and clinically normal child suggest that the child is uninfected. The disappearance of maternal antibodies should be monitored and confirmed once negative. On present knowledge, children who are antibody-negative on at least two samples and are clinically well can be considered to be uninfected.[18]

Natural history

Children may develop a wide range of manifestations of HIV disease, which depend in part on exposure to different infections, and treatment and care

Table 5.3 Natural history of vertically acquired paediatric HIV infection

- Some 25–30% of children develop AIDS in the first year of life, most commonly *Pneumocystis carinii* pneumonia
- Lymphocytic interstitial pneumonitis is frequent, but often asymptomatic
- Primary, rather than reactivation of, opportunistic infections occurs. (Cytomegalovirus, retinitis and *Toxoplasmosis* are rare.)
- Bacterial infections are common, particularly with *Streptococcus pneumoniae* and *Haemophilus influenzae*
- The presenting pattern of encephalopathy varies with age
- Growth failure occurs in addition to failure to thrive
- Kaposi's sarcoma is rare, but lymphomas (especially central nervous system) occur

available in different parts of the world (Table 5.3). The initial presentation is often non-specific and includes generalized lymphadenopathy, hepato-splenomegaly, diarrhoea, fever unexplained by other causes, failure to thrive and parotitis. Without a definitive diagnosis of HIV infection it may not be possible to determine whether these symptoms or signs are HIV-related, particularly in populations with a high background prevalence of intercurrent infections. The clinical spectrum of paediatric HIV infection is described in the classification of HIV in children developed by Centers for Disease Control, Atlanta, USA in 1987.[19] The definition of paediatric AIDS includes the following AIDS defining events: opportunistic infections; recurrent severe bacterial infections; failure to thrive; encephalopathy; malignancy and lymphoid interstitial pneumonitis (LIP). LIP is often asymptomatic (diagnosed on chest X-ray only), is not associated with a poor prognosis, and should probably be excluded from the definition of paediatric AIDS.

In the developing world, severe failure to thrive with diarrhoea, bacterial infections, measles and tuberculosis are frequent in HIV-infected children and have a high mortality.[20]

In Europe,[18] based on follow-up from birth, the initial clinical manifestations in symptomatic infected children were a combination of persistent lymphadenopathy, hepatomegaly and splenomegaly, although in 30% of these children the initial presentation was AIDS or oral *Candida* rapidly leading on to AIDS. Using survival methods, this study showed that an estimated 83% of infected children exhibited signs of HIV infection within 6 months of age, whether hypergammaglobulinaemia, clinical signs, or a low CD4:CD8 ratio. By 12 months, 26% had developed AIDS and 17% had died of HIV-related disease. This is very similar to the rates reported from the Swiss perinatal study.[7] The rate of progression of HIV disease declined after 12 months, and the condition of most children remained stable or even improved over the second year. The clinical manifestations and the progression of the disease were closely related to the immunological status of the child; for example, neurological problems became apparent only when the immune system was depressed and were not usually presenting symptoms. In the Italian Register, which includes both children followed from birth and those presenting with HIV-related manifestations, 70% were alive at 6 years and 50% at 9 years.[5]

CHILDREN WITH AIDS

Several studies have described the spectrum of AIDS in children either from hospital-based cohorts,[21,22] or population-based through surveillance systems.[2,23] The most common AIDS indicator disease in the first year of life is *Pneumocystis carinii* pneumonia (PCP) which has a high mortality.[21,22,24,25] Children surviving PCP often develop subsequent AIDS defining events, particularly HIV encephalopathy.[21] Children more frequently develop bacterial infections than HIV-infected adults.[26] LIP is common in children with vertically acquired HIV, but is rare in adults and older children with haemophilia and HIV. Kaposi sarcoma is rare in children but lymphoma (most frequently central nervous system lymphoma) is increasingly being reported.

Opportunistic infections

In Europe and the USA, PCP is the most commonly reported AIDS defining event and occurs most frequently in the first 6 months of life.[2,24,25] The CD4 count is not necessarily predictive of the imminent onset of PCP. PCP has a high mortality, even if intensive care, high-dose trimethoprim-sulphamethoxazole (TMP–SMX) and steroids are used for treatment.[24,25] One of the authors (Gibb) has observed that in two-thirds of cases of PCP in the British Isles, PCP in the infant was the first indication of HIV infection in a family where the mother was unaware of her HIV status. Children recovering from PCP soon develop other AIDS defining events, in particular HIV encephalopathy, and the overall survival is poor.[21,22]

Other opportunistic infections such as oral and perineal *Candida* are common. However, toxoplasmosis and cryptococcal meningitis are rare in children. Cytomegalovirus (CMV) may cause disseminated disease, most frequently in the first months of life, but retinitis is unusual. As in adults, CMV is often cultured from asymptomatic children with or without HIV infection, and it may be difficult to define its role in the pathogenesis of symptoms. Cryptosporidial diarrhoea and infections with atypical mycobacteria are being diagnosed with increasing frequency in children with profound immune deficiency.

Bacterial infections

HIV-infected children are prone to a wide range of bacterial infections. The organisms most frequently responsible are polysaccharide encapsulated bacteria, e.g. *Streptococcus pneumoniae* and *Haemophilus influenzae*, *Salmonella* species.[27] AIDS is diagnosed when two serious bacterial infections (pneumonia, meningitis, septicaemia, osteomyelitis and cellulitis) occur within a 2-year period. In a large multicentre American study of intravenous immunoglobulin (IVIG) therapy in children with HIV infection, 40% of infections presented as pneumonia, which occurred more frequently than in normal children or in adults with HIV infections.[27] This study showed that IVIG therapy may provide some protection against a wide range of bacterial and viral infections. Given monthly at a dose of 0.4 g/kg, it approximately halved the incidence of bacterial infections, but there was no effect on mortality. Further research is needed to identify those children who would benefit from IVIG therapy. TMP–SMX prophylaxis, used to prevent PCP (see below) has also been shown to provide some protection against bacterial infections, both in adults with HIV infection and in children with leukaemia.[28] As regular insertion of intravenous cannulae causes discomfort and IVIG therapy is expensive, IVIG could be reserved for those children who suffer from recurrent bacterial infections despite daily TMP–SMX prophylaxis. Immunizations against *H. influenzae* and *S. pneumoniae* are recommended for all infected children, and should be given early in the course of HIV infection as their efficacy in children with severe immune suppression is much reduced.

Failure to thrive

The causes of failure to thrive in HIV infection are multifactorial and include inadequate nutritional intake secondary to poor appetite, oral infections or neurological disease; malabsorption resulting from HIV enteropathy itself or bacterial colonization of the small intestine; and increased nutritional requirements as a result of recurrent infections. Early attention to nutrition, with supplementation and nasogastric feeding as required, is important. In addition to the severe failure to thrive observed in young children, as children with HIV infection live longer, poor growth is being increasingly observed.[29] Hormonal factors may also play a role in its pathogenesis.

HIV encephalopathy

This presents with developmental delay or loss of milestones in young children, impairment of expressive language over receptive language in the 2–4-year-old child, and behavioural abnormalities with loss of concentration and memory in the older child. Progressive motor signs, particularly spastic diplegia and oral motor dysfunction, are a marked feature, particularly in the early-onset encephalopathy.[30] Acquired microcephaly in these children may be accompanied by cerebral atrophy or calcification within the basal ganglia as shown on computed tomography or magnetic resonance scan. Rarer conditions such as cerebral abscess, toxoplasmosis or lymphoma should be excluded.

It may be difficult to differentiate signs of early encephalopathy from poor functioning due to chronic illness and poor social and emotional circumstances, particularly in the older child. Therefore regular monitoring of the child's neurodevelopment is an important part of management for children with HIV infection.

Lymphocytic interstitial pneumonitis

This slowly progressive, chronic lung disease of unknown aetiology may affect up to 40% of children vertically infected with HIV but is rare in adults or older children with haemophilia and HIV.[31] It is characterized by bilateral fine nodular infiltrates on chest X-ray, and histology shows infiltration of the interstitium with small lymphocytes and plasma cells. Despite marked abnormalities on chest X-ray, the child may be asymptomatic with no abnormal findings on auscultation. Although cough, shortness of breath, hypoxaemia and digital clubbing may develop with time, children rarely die of LIP alone. A presumptive diagnosis may be made from clinical features and chest X-ray appearance, after other causes of interstitial pneumonia have been excluded. This may be difficult as LIP may coexist with tuberculosis, bacterial lung infections and PCP. A definitive diagnosis can be made by lung biopsy.

   Management consists of making the diagnosis early and it is useful to do a chest X-ray on all children at the time of diagnosis of HIV infection and then yearly in asymptomatic children. Children may be asymptomatic with no change in X-ray appearances for many years but may eventually start to develop secondary bacterial chest infections and bronchiectasis. Although there are no data to support its use in early asymptomatic LIP, zidovudine has been reported to be helpful in chronic symptomatic LIP. Steroids may also be of benefit in severely symptomatic LIP, although their effect is often only temporary.[32]

OTHER ASPECTS OF MANAGEMENT

The frequency of follow-up by the paediatrician will depend upon the child's symptoms, the need for treatment, social circumstances and the degree of medical and social support provided by other agencies (Table 5.4).

Pneumocystis carinii prophylaxis

TMP–SMX (co-trimoxazole, Septrin) is the drug of choice, and is well-tolerated by children. The dose is 150 mg/m^2 trimethoprim, 750 mg/m^2 sulphamethoxazole given daily or three times weekly. Guidelines for prophylaxis based on the CD4 count have been published by Centers for Disease Control, Atlanta.[33] However, this requires frequent CD4 measurements, and will not identify those children who develop PCP very early or suddenly between visits. It has been suggested by some paediatricians therefore to consider giving prophylaxis to all HIV-infected children, irrespective of their CD4 count, and to give it to children of indeterminate HIV infection status

Table 5.4 Key issues in management

In pregnancy
  Advice about breast-feeding and follow-up of the child
First month
  Early diagnosis
  Immunizations
  Regular clinical and immunological monitoring
Prophylaxis against infections
  Pneumocystis carinii pneumonia
  Bacterial infections
Antiretroviral therapy
  Zidovudine
  Dideoxyinosine
  Combination therapy
Rapid treatment of complications
Attention to nutrition
Early identification of developmental problems
Family-centred medical, social and psychological care

in the early weeks of life if close follow-up is difficult. Further research is required to evaluate the cost and benefit of the Centers for Disease Control and other prophylaxis regimens for children born to HIV-positive women. Dapsone, at a dose of 1 mg/kg per day, may be used for children who develop allergic reactions to co-trimoxazole. Phase I studies of monthly pentamidine 300 mg via a Respigard nebulizer are currently in progress in the USA.

Immunizations

Children infected with HIV should receive all immunizations with the exception of BCG, which should be withheld from those with symptomatic disease and from all children where tuberculosis prevalence is low (Table 5.5). There have been no reports of an increased number of adverse reactions to live vaccines, although some paediatricians may prefer to use killed polio, because of the theoretical risk of transmission of live polio virus to other immunocompromised family members. Infected children should receive zoster immune globulin or hyperimmune globulin after exposure to chickenpox or measles respectively. It has been demonstrated that asymptomatic children with HIV infection produce satisfactory antibody responses to measles vaccination but these may decrease with declining immune function.[34] With decreasing immunocompetence in the HIV-infected child, it may be prudent to give booster immunizations, for example against measles.

Table 5.5 Immunizations

Efficacy is better in early disease
Live vaccines appear to be safe
Locally recommended schedule should be followed

Antiretroviral drugs

Zidovudine (ZDV; 3'azido-3'deoxythymidine; AZT) is a nucleoside analogue with in vitro inhibitory effects against HIV. In adults with AIDS or symptomatic HIV infection, ZDV is associated with prolongation of survival.[35] Use of the drug in asymptomatic adults suggests it may reduce the progression rate to AIDS by up to 50% in the short term, although its effect in the long term and also its effect on survival await the outcome of other studies.[35,36] No efficacy studies have been performed in children, although data from open labelled studies suggest benefit in children with symptomatic HIV disease, particularly in those with encephalopathy.[37,38] It is not clear when treatment with zidovudine should be initiated in children with early or asymptomatic disease and practice varies widely. In an attempt to answer this question two trials of early versus deferred treatment in asymptomatic disease have recently started in Europe and the USA. The recommended dose of ZDV for children is 600–720 mg/m^2 per day in three to four divided doses. However, a study comparing this with lower doses is ongoing in the USA as it may be that, as in adults, a lower dose is adequate. Zidovudine can cause a reduction in neutrophil count and haemoglobin concentration, and a full blood count should be checked regularly, particularly in the first weeks of therapy. Haematological toxicity is, however, reversible. Of concern has been the identification of in vitro resistance to ZDV, developing particularly fast in patients with more advanced disease. Thus, monotherapy of this drug is likely to be of only limited value in delaying disease progression in the long term.

2', 3' dideoxyinosine (didanosine, DDi) is another nucleoside analogue with in vitro activity against HIV. In adults who have already received ZDV, switching to DDi resulted in slower progression of disease in the short term compared with remaining on ZDV alone. However in a large trial of DDi in adults with late-stage disease in Europe (ALPHA trial), preliminary results showed no clinical or survival benefit in those taking DDi 750 mg/day compared with 200 mg/day, although there was a significantly greater rise in CD4 count in those taking the higher dose.[39] Adverse reactions to DDi, which include pancreatitis, peripheral neuropathy and hepatic dysfunction, are related both to daily and cumulative dose administered. A phase II study of DDi in children showed similar results to those observed in adults.[40] DDi has been licensed in the USA and some European countries and is already being used in children with intolerance and apparent resistance to ZDV. Its efficiency compared to ZDV monotherapy remains unclear and studies comparing it with combination therapy (AZT and DDi) are planned in Europe. Other combinations of antiretroviral drugs (e.g. ZDV and dideoxycytosine or DDc) are currently being evaluated in adults. In the future, combinations or sequential use of different antiretroviral drugs are likely to be the most effective and least toxic way of treating HIV infection and studies must be set up in children in parallel with those being undertaken in adults.

Support for the whole family

Coping with the complex psychological and social needs of the family is one of the most important and challenging aspects of paediatric HIV management. The child may be the first family member to be diagnosed and parents may have to face the prospect of being tested for HIV at a time when their child is seriously ill. Mothers feel an enormous sense of guilt at having infected their own child, and often focus on the child's needs at the expense of their own health. There is still tremendous stigma attached to a diagnosis of HIV, and families often feel socially and culturally isolated. Illness and unemployment can create financial problems. It is important to establish links with key support agencies in the community, while also respecting the family's need for confidentiality.

The management of paediatric HIV involves the clinician in a wide range of medical, social and psychological problems. For this reason, HIV-infected children and their families are best supported by a multidisciplinary team of health professionals who can deliver coordinated care in a family-oriented, child-centred manner. Helping HIV-infected children and their families lead healthier, happier lives must be one of the biggest and most rewarding challenges of paediatrics.

KEY POINTS FOR CLINICAL PRACTICE

- The rate of mother-to-child transmission in Europe is about 15%.
- Transmission is associated with progression of disease, gestation less than 34 weeks and breast-feeding.
- The early diagnosis of HIV infection in a child of an HIV-infected mother may be difficult.
- The initial presentation of HIV disease is often non-specific, although about 30% of infected children present with AIDS.
- The most common AIDS indicator disease is *Pneumocystis carinii* pneumonia, usually occurring in the first 6 months of life, with a high mortality.
- Co-trimoxazole may be used as prophylaxis against *Pneumocystis carinii* pneumonia.
- Prophylactic intravenous immunoglobulin therapy may confer some protection against a wide range of bacterial infections, as may co-trimoxazole.
- Immunization against *Haemophilus influenzae* and *Streptococcus pneumoniae* is recommended for all infected children.
- Lymphocytic interstitial pneumonitis may affect up to 40% of vertically infected children, but is often asymptomatic.
- It is not clear when treatment with zidovudine should be initiated in children with early or asymptomatic disease.

REFERENCES

1 Chin J. Epidemiology. Current and future dimensions of the HIV/AIDS pandemic in women and children. Lancet 1990; 336: 221–224

2 World Health Organization/EC Collaborating Centre on AIDS. AIDS surveillance in Europe. WHO quarterly report no 35. Saint-Maurice, France, WHO, 1992: 4–24

3 Editorial. The 'silent' legacy of AIDS: children who survive their parents and siblings. JAMA 1992; 268: 3478–3479

4 Berkley S, Naamara W, Okware S et al. AIDS and HIV infection in Uganda — are more women infected than men? AIDS 1990; 4: 1237–1242

5 Tovo P, De Martino M, Gabiano C, Cappello N, D'Elia E and Italian register for HIV infection in children. Prognostic factors and survival in children with perinatal HIV-1 infection. Lancet 1992; 339: 1249–1253

6 Lynn R, Hall SM. The British Paediatric Surveillance Unit: activities and developments in 1990 and 1991. Communicable Disease Report 1992; 2: R145–R148.

7 Kind C, Brandle B, Wyler C-A et al. Swiss Neonatal HIV Study Group Epidemiology of vertically transmitted HIV-1 infection in Switzerland: results of a nationwide prospective study. Eur J Pediatr 1992; 151: 442–448

8 Ades AE, Davison CF, Holland FJ et al Vertically transmitted HIV infection in the Bristish Isles. Br Med J 1993; 306: 1296–1299

9 Schoenbaum EE, Davenny K, Selwyn PA. The impact of pregnancy on HIV-related disease. In: Hudson CN, Sharp F, eds. AIDS and obstetrics and gynaecology. London: Royal College of Obstetricians and Gynaecologists, 1988: pp 65–75

10 Newell ML, Peckham C. Risk factors for vertical transmission of HIV-1 and early markers of HIV-1 infection in children. AIDS 1993; 7(suppl 1): 591–597

11 European Collaborative Study. Risk factors for mother-to-child transmission of HIV-1. Lancet 1992; 339: 1007–1012

12 Consensus workshop, Siena, Italy. Maternal factors involved in mother-to-child transmission of HIV-1. J AIDS 1992; 5: 1019–1029

13 Gabiano C, Tovo P, de Martino M et al. Mother-to-child transmission of human immunodeficiency virus type 1: risk of infection and correlates of transmission. Pediatrics 1992; 90: 369–374

14 Dunn D, Newell M, Ades A, Peckham C. Risk of human immunodeficiency virus type 1 transmission through breastfeeding. Lancet 1992; 340: 585–588

15 Consensus Workshop Siena, Italy. Early diagnosis of HIV infection in infants. J AIDS 1992; 5: 1169–1178

16 Burgard M, Mayaux M-J, Blanche BAS et al. The use of viral culture and p24 antigen testing to diagnose human immunodeficiency virus infection in neonates. N Engl J Med 1992; 327: 1192–1197

17 Miles SA, Balden E, Magpantay L et al. Rapid serologic testing with immune-complex dissociated HIV p24 antigen for early detection of HIV infection in neonates. N Engl J Med 1993; 328: 297–302

18 European Collaborative Study. Children born to women with HIV-1 infection: natural history and risk of transmission. Lancet 1991; 337: 253–260

19 Centers for Disease Control. Classification system for human immunodeficiency virus (HIV) infection in children under 13 years of age. Morbid Mortal Week Rep 1987; 15: 225–236

20 Pavia AT, Long EG, Ryder RW et al. Diarrhea among African children born to human immunodeficiency virus 1-infected mothers: clinical, microbiologic and epidemiologic features. Pediatr Infect Dis J 1992; 11: 996–1003

21 Blanche S, Tardieu M, Duliege A et al. Longitudinal study of 94 symptomatic infants with perinatally acquired human immunodeficiency virus infection. Am J Dis Child 1990; 144: 1210–1215

22 Scott GB, Hutto C, Makuch RW et al. Survival in children with perinatally acquired human immunodeficiency virus type 1 infection. N Engl J Med 1989; 321: 1791–1796

23 Thomas P, Singh T, Williams R, Blum S. Trends in survival for children reported with maternally transmitted acquired immunodeficiency syndrome in New York City, 1982 to 1989. Pediatr Infect Dis J 1992; 11: 34–39

24 Connor E, Bagarazzi M, McSherry G et al. Clinical and laboratory correlates of

Pneumocystis carinii pneumonia in children infected with HIV. JAMA 1991; 265: 1693–1697

25 Vernon DD, Holzman BH, Lewis P, Scott GB, Birriel JA, Scott MB. Respiratory failure in children with acquired immunodeficiency syndrome and acquired immunodeficiency syndrome-related complex. Pediatrics 1988; 83: 223–228

26 The National Institute of Child Health and Human Development Intravenous Immunoglobulin Study Group. Intravenous immune globulin for the prevention of bacterial infections in children with symptomatic human immunodeficiency virus infection. N Engl J Med 1991; 325: 73–80

27 Mofenson LM, Moye J, Bethel J, Hirschhorn R, Jordan C, Nugent R. Prophylactic intravenous immunoglobulin in HIV-infected children with CD4 + counts of 0.20×10^9/L or more. JAMA 1992; 268: 483–488

28 Hughes WT. *Pneumocystis carinii* pneumonia: new approaches to diagnosis, treatment and prevention. Pediatr Infect Dis J 1991; 10: 391–399

29 Laue L, Cutler GB. Neuroendocrine and growth dysfunction. In: Pizzo PA, Wilfert CM, eds Pediatric AIDS: the challenge of HIV infection in infants, children and adolescents. Baltimore: Williams & Wilkins, 1991: pp 407–419

30 European Collaborative Study. Neurological signs in young children with HIV infection. Pediatr Infect Dis J 1990; 9: 402–406

31 Jones P. HIV infection and haemophilia. Arch Dis Child 1990; 65: 364–368

32 Connor EM, Marquis J, Oleske JM. Lymphoid interstitial pneumonitis. In: Pizzo PA, Wilfert CM, eds. Pediatric AIDS: the challenge of HIV infection in infants, children and adolescents. Baltimore: Williams & Wilkins, 1991: pp 343–354

33 Centers for Disease Control. Guidelines for prophylaxis against *Pneumocystis carinii* pneumonia for children infected with human immunodeficiency virus. JAMA 1991; 265: 1637–1644

34 Lepage P, Dabis F, Msellati P et al. Safety and immunogenicity of high-dose Edmonston-Zagreb measles vaccine in children with HIV-1 infection. Am J Dis Child 1992; 146: 550–555

35 Hamilton JD, Hartigan PM, Simberkoff MS et al. A controlled trial of early versus late treatment with zidovudine in symptomatic human immunodeficiency virus infection — results of the Veterans Affairs Cooperative Study. N Eng J Med 1992; 326: 437–443

36 Volberding PA, Lagakos SW, Koch MA et al. Zidovudine in asymptomatic human immunodeficiency virus infection. N Engl J Med 1990; 322: 941–949

37 Pizzo PA, Eddy J, Falloon J et al. Effect of continuous intravenous infusion of zidovudine (AZT) in children with symptomatic HIV infection. N Engl J Med 1988; 319: 889–896

38 McKinney RE, Maha MA, Connor EM et al. A multicenter trial of oral zidovudine in children with advanced human immunodeficiency virus disease. N Eng J Med 1991; 324: 1018–1025

39 Darbyshire JH, Aboulker JP. Didanosine for zidovudine-intolerant patients with HIV disease. Lancet 1992; 340: 1346–1347

40 Butler KM, Husson RN, Balis FM et al. Dideoxyinosine in children with symptomatic human immunodeficiency virus infection. N Engl J Med 1991; 324: 137–144

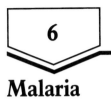

Malaria

B. Greenwood

Malaria remains one of the most important human infections. It is estimated that approximately 500 million clinical attacks of malaria occur each year and that malaria causes 0.5–2 million deaths a year.[1] Most of these deaths occur among children in Africa. Unfortunately, the global malaria situation is deteriorating. In many tropical African countries the number of children admitted to hospital with malaria is increasing and, in the Far East, parasites have been isolated recently which are resistant to almost all antimalarial drugs.

EPIDEMIOLOGY

Four species of malaria parasite infect humans — *Plasmodium falciparum, P. malariae, P. vivax* and *P. ovale.* The life cycle of *P. falciparum* is shown in Figure. 6.1. The life cycles of *P. vivax* and *P. ovale* differ from *P. falciparum* in that these parasites have a secondary liver cycle that can lead to relapses.

Infections caused by *P. falciparum* are the most dangerous because this parasite can sequester in small blood vessels and thus cause serious complications such as cerebral malaria. *P. malariae* does not sequester but may occasionally cause chronic renal damage. *P. vivax* rarely causes serious complications.

Malaria is still endemic throughout most of the tropics and its range extends north of the tropics in Asia. In colder areas *P. vivax* is the dominant parasite. Within malaria endemic areas the risk of infection may vary substantially from area to area. Thus, in the case of Thailand, visitors to Bangkok are at minimal risk of malaria whilst the risk for visitors to areas bordering Burma or Cambodia is high. In many areas, malaria transmission is seasonal so that the risk of infection varies with the time of year.

PATHOLOGY AND PATHOGENESIS

Malaria fever

Peaks of malaria fever coincide with the rupture of parasitized red blood cells (PRBC), strongly suggesting that a pyrogenic malaria 'toxin' is released into

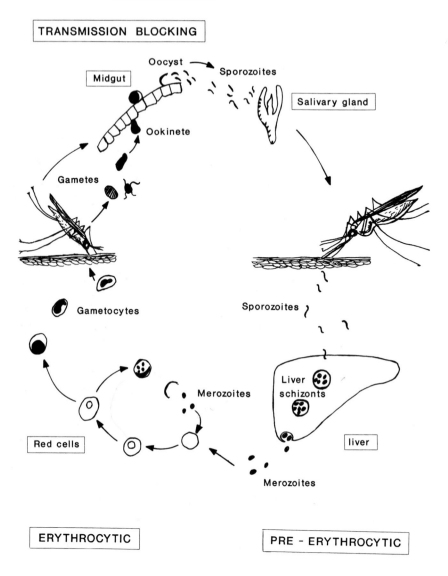

Fig. 6.1   The life cycle of *Plasmodium falciparum* and stages of the cycle at which vaccine-induced immunity is directed.

the circulation at that time. Recent studies suggest that the factor involved is a glycolipid.[2,3] The malaria toxin is not a direct pyrogen and there is strong evidence that it acts by stimulating host mononuclear cells to produce pyrogenic cytokines such as tumour necrosis factor (TNF). Thus, it has been shown that a peak production of TNF coincides with schizont rupture in in vitro culture experiments and that peak plasma levels of TNF are found at the onset of fever paroxysms in patients infected with *P. vivax*.[4] Furthermore, the fever of children with *P. falciparum* malaria can be suppressed by administration of an anti-TNF monoclonal antibody.[5]

Cerebral malaria

Postmortem examinations of patients who have died of cerebral malaria usually show small cerebral vessels packed with PRBC, which frequently contain mature schizonts. Electron-dense knobs are present on the surface of PRBC close to their points of contact with endothelial cells. These histological changes suggest strongly that adherence of PRBC to the endothelium of cerebral vessels is an essential part of the pathogenesis of cerebral malaria. The mechanism of this interaction is currently an area of intensive research. Because of the difficulty of experimental work with cerebral vessels, most of the studies that have been done so far have used human umbilical vein endothelial cells or melanoma cell lines.[6] At least three receptors for parasite adhesion have been identified on the surface of target cells — thrombospondin, CD36 and ICAM-1 — but the involvement of additional receptors is suspected. Wild parasites vary in their ability to bind to each of these receptors but no consistent association has been found between the ability of parasites to bind to an individual receptor and their ability to cause cerebral malaria.

A strong contender for the ligand on the surface of red blood cells (RBC) infected with *P. falciparum* is Pf EMP-1, a large molecular weight protein found on the surface of infected RBC.[7] The structure of Pf EMP-1 varies between isolates and true antigenic variation of the protein has been demonstrated during the course of in vitro culture of a cloned parasite.[8] Thus, development of a vaccine based on this protein will be difficult. Another binding site on the surface of infected RBC is a region of the structural protein, band 3, which is conformationally altered in some way as a result of malaria infection of the RBC.[6] PRBC bind to non-infected RBC to form clusters of infected and non-infected RBC known as rosettes. Parasites obtained from Gambian children with cerebral malaria formed rosettes more readily than did parasites obtained from children with mild malaria,[9] suggesting a role for rosettes in the pathogenesis of cerebral malaria. However, it is possible that an ability to form rosettes is a phenotypic marker for some other parasite characteristic which is associated with virulence. Two parasite proteins thought to be involved in rosette formation have been identified. PRBC form rosettes more readily with RBC of blood group A or B than with RBC of blood group O,[10] so that it is likely that the ABO blood group polysaccharide is involved in some way with rosette formation.

Other recent studies suggest a completely different mechanism for the pathogenesis of cerebral malaria. High levels of the cytokine TNF have been found in the plasma of patients with cerebral malaria, especially in those who subsequently died.[11,12] However, not all patients with cerebral malaria have high levels of TNF and high TNF levels are found also during fever paroxysms in patients infected with *P. vivax*, who do not develop cerebral malaria.[4] Thus, it seems unlikely that TNF alone can cause cerebral malaria.

Cytokines such as TNF can upregulate the expression of ICAM-1 and of other receptors on the surface of endothelial cells,[13] so a model can be developed of how these two different pathological processes might interact to produce cerebral malaria (Fig. 6.2). Initial adherence of PRBC to the surface of an endothelial cell followed by schizont rupture might lead to local production of TNF, upregulation of endothelial receptors, binding of further PRBC to adjacent endothelial cells, further release of TNF and a vicious circle resulting finally in obstruction to the circulation through the affected vessel.

A further twist to this complicated story has been added by the recent observation that TNF upregulates nitric oxide synthetase activity. Thus, it is possible that large amounts of nitric oxide are produced locally at sites of sequestered parasites. It has been suggested that this nitric oxide diffuses across the wall of the affected cerebral vessel into the brain where it interferes with the activity of calcium influx mechanisms, inducing coma in a manner analogous to some anaesthetics.[14]

Anaemia

Severe anaemia can result from direct destruction of large numbers of RBC by the parasite. However, severe anaemia may occur also in patients with only low levels of parasitaemia; in such patients it has a more complex pathogenesis. Non-infected as well as infected RBC are destroyed more rapidly than normal in patients with malaria.[15] This probably results from both increased reticuloendothelial cell activity and from accelerated red cell clearance following the deposition of both immunoglobulin and complement components on the surface of infected and non-infected RBC, although the importance of the latter mechanism is disputed. Bone marrow biopsies taken from some children with malaria show dyserythropoiesis.[16] Thus, both enhanced destruction of non-infected and infected RBC and diminished production of RBC are likely to contribute to the anaemia of malaria.

NATURALLY ACQUIRED IMMUNITY TO MALARIA

It is doubtful whether complete immunity to malaria is ever achieved as a result of natural infection, for adults exposed to malaria throughout their life continue to have occasional episodes of asymptomatic infection. However, repeated exposure to infection leads, after a few years, to the acquisition of immunity against clinical malaria, in particular to protection against severe disease. Continued exposure to malaria parasites is required to maintain this immunity. How is this naturally acquired immunity to malaria achieved?

Early studies showed that plasma from immune, adult Gambians reduced parasitaemia in infected children,[17] indicating that humoral factors, probably antibody, are involved in naturally acquired immunity to malaria. This view is supported by the fact that infants are protected against severe clinical

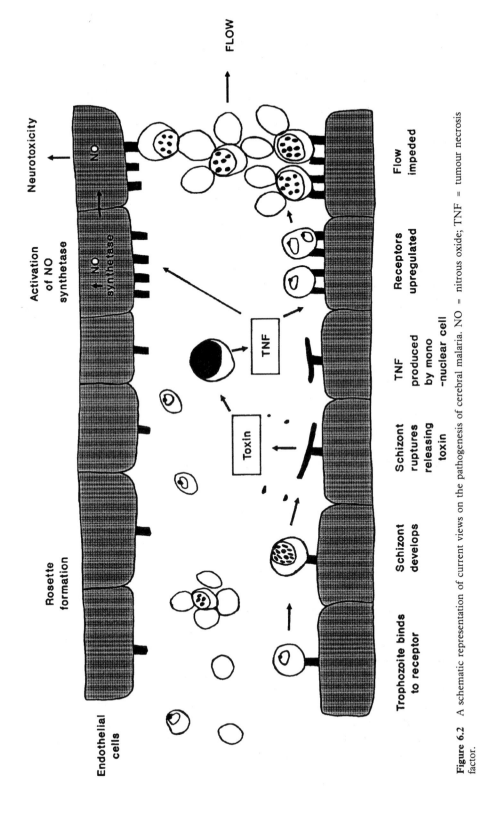

Figure 6.2 A schematic representation of current views on the pathogenesis of cerebral malaria. NO = nitrous oxide; TNF = tumour necrosis factor.

malaria for several months after birth, probably by maternal antibody transferred across the placenta.

Defining which antibody or antibodies are the most important mediators of protective humoral immunity has been difficult and it seems unlikely that any one antibody has a dominant role. Perhaps different individuals achieve protection using different antibodies dependent upon their human leukocyte antigen (HLA) class II genotype. Careful epidemiological studies in endemic areas have provided some evidence that antibodies to epitopes of the *P. falciparum* blood stage antigens RESA and MSP1 are associated with some protection against clinical malaria,[18] but these effects have not been marked.

The contribution of cell-mediated immune responses to the acquisition of protective immunity to malaria in humans has not been clearly defined. Proliferative and cytokine responses to many malaria antigens have been demonstrated in immune individuals but these do not correlate directly with protective immunity.[19] It is of interest that no clear evidence has been found that human immunodeficiency virus (HIV) infection, despite its deleterious effect on CD4 cells, reduces resistance to malaria. It is likely that the tests that have been used to investigate cell-mediated immune responses in malaria-immune subjects so far have been too crude to be instructive and that more detailed studies of the responses of individual T-cell subsets will be needed to define more accurately the role of cell-mediated immune responses in protection against this infection.

Irradiated sporozoite vaccines probably achieve their protective effect by inducing cytotoxic T cells which attack parasite-infected liver cells. Thus, the possibility has been raised that such cells might play an important part in establishing naturally acquired immunity. This idea is supported by the recent demonstration of cytotoxic T cells reacting against liver stage and sporozoite antigens in some adult residents of malaria-endemic areas.[20]

CLINICAL FEATURES

The spectrum of clinical malaria

Malaria can vary in severity from an asymptomatic infection to an illness which kills within a few hours of the first onset of symptoms. Severe disease

Table 6.1 WHO criteria for defining severe malaria in children [23]

Cerebral malaria (unrousable coma)
Severe normocytic anaemia (haemoglobin <5 g/dl, parasitaemia >10 000/μl)
Renal failure (urine output <12 ml/kg per 24 h + creatinine >265 μmol/l)
Pulmonary oedema
Hypoglycaemia (whole blood glucose <2.2 mmol/l)
Circulatory collapse (systolic blood pressure <50 mm/Hg + cold extremities)
Spontaneous bleeding and/or disseminated intravascular coagulation
Repeated, generalized convulsions
Acidaemia (arterial pH <7.25) or acidosis (plasma bicarbonate <15 mmol/l)
Malaria haemoglobinuria (not drug-induced)

is more likely during a first attack of malaria than in subsequent attacks but the level of prior exposure to malaria is not the only determinant of severity. In populations where malaria is highly endemic only a small proportion of children, usually about 1–2%, develop severe disease.[21] Both parasite and host genetic factors, such as haemoglobin and HLA class I and class II genotypes, appear to be important in defining this at-risk group.[22]

Uncomplicated malaria

Fever is the characteristic clinical feature of malaria and few patients do not have fever or a past history of recent fever. Fever may be intermittent, with rigors and sweating, but frequently a history of persistent fever is obtained. Patients usually complain of other non-specific symptoms such as headache, nausea and myalgia, all of which may be severe. Febrile convulsions may occur in young children. Occasionally, gastrointestinal or respiratory symptoms predominate.

A child with malaria is usually febrile, although the temperature is occasionally normal or subnormal, for example after a paroxysm. The conjunctivae may be pale. The spleen may be enlarged and tender, especially if the illness has been present for a number of days or if the child has been exposed previously to malaria. Rupture of the spleen is a rare complication which has been described most frequently in patients infected with *P. vivax*. Slight enlargement and tenderness of the liver are found more consistently than splenomegaly. The respiratory rate may be raised and occasional crepitations and rhonchi may be heard. There may be some degree of normocytic anaemia; thrombocytopenia and a polymorphonuclear neutrophil leukocytosis are frequently found.

Severe malaria

A number of complications of malaria have been used to define severe malaria (Table 6.1).[23] In non-immune adults, severe malaria is usually characterized by involvement of several organs. Thus, cerebral malaria, acute renal failure, liver failure, pulmonary oedema and peripheral circulatory collapse may be encountered in various combinations. Bleeding associated with disseminated intravascular coagulation may occur. This is the usual picture of severe malaria seen in residents of South-East Asia and in expatriate visitors to malaria-endemic areas. In contrast, in tropical Africa, most children who satisfy the diagnostic criteria for severe malaria have cerebral malaria, severe anaemia, generalized convulsions or hypoglycaemia.

Cerebral malaria is the most serious complication of *P. falciparum* infection. Loss of consciousness can occur with frightening rapidity and some children are already in deep coma by the time they reach hospital. Fits are frequent and status epilepticus may occur. A modification of the Glasgow Coma Score is useful in categorizing the level of coma in African children with cerebral malaria.[24] Localizing neurological signs are found infrequently but in severe cases there may be increased muscle tone, opisthotonus, posturing and features of decerebrate rigidity. Papilloedema is rare but retinal haemorrhages are sometimes seen. Lumbar puncture may show a modest increase in cerebrospinal fluid pressure and raised intracranial pressure has been confirmed in a small number of Kenyan children with cerebral malaria using an intracranial manometer. For this reason some paediatricians do not recommend lumbar puncture in children with suspected cerebral malaria[25] but, if this advice is followed, antibiotics must be given as well as antimalarials as it is not always possible to differentiate cerebral malaria from meningitis on clinical grounds.

The prognosis of cerebral malaria is poor, even under optimal conditions of care. Mortality in children ranges from 10 to 30% depending upon the initial coma score. High initial TNF and blood lactate levels indicate a poor prognosis. Deaths from cerebral malaria usually occur within the first 24 h of admission to hospital but occasional, late deaths are encountered. The cause of death is not always obvious but, in some cases, respiratory arrest has been observed. Some children make a rapid and progressive recovery but deterioration in conscious level and recurrent episodes of convulsions and hypoglycaemia may occur after an initial period of apparent improvement. Above 10% of survivors are left with obvious neurological sequelae such as aphasia, a hemiplegia or cortical blindness.[26] An unusual cerebellar syndrome has been described after malaria in India and Sri Lanka. It is likely that survivors from cerebral malaria are left with minor neurological deficits but the frequency with which these occur is not known.

Severe anaemia may occur as part of an acute malaria illness associated with high levels of parasitaemia and massive destruction of RBC, but it may also present as a more insidious illness associated with persistent low levels of parasitaemia. This latter form of malaria anaemia is common in areas with moderate levels of chloroquine resistance, where chloroquine treatment controls acute symptoms of malaria whilst allowing persistence of a chronic parasitaemia and the slow development of anaemia. There are no special clinical features characteristic of malaria anaemia; children frequently present in heart failure.

Severe hypoglycaemia is found in a proportion of children with severe malaria and hypoglycaemia may be exacerbated by treatment with quinine. Other forms of severe malaria such as renal failure, liver failure or pulmonary oedema are seen only rarely in African children. There is little recent information about the clinical spectrum of falciparum malaria in children in other parts of the world. However, a recent study has shown that renal failure and jaundice are more common in Vietnamese children with severe malaria than in African children with this condition.[27]

Late complications of malaria

Septicaemia, often caused by a *Salmonella* species, may follow an acute attack of malaria, especially among patients with anaemia. A small proportion of *P. malariae* infections are followed by an immune complex-mediated nephritis which usually presents as the nephrotic syndrome. This frequently progresses to chronic renal failure and death.

DIAGNOSIS

There are no clinical features diagnostic of uncomplicated malaria, so the infection must be considered in the differential diagnosis of any febrile child resident in a malaria-endemic area or in any such child who has been a recent visitor to such an area, even if chemoprophylaxis has been taken. Similarly, cerebral malaria must be considered as a possible diagnosis in any such child who fits or develops impairment of consciousness. Failure to elicit a history of a recent visit to a malaria-endemic area may be fatal.

Many children with malaria have respiratory symptoms and a raised respiratory rate and so risk being misdiagnosed as a case of pneumonia, especially by primary health care workers who are taught to diagnose pneumonia on the basis of cough and a raised respiratory rate.

Diagnosis of malaria is established by detection of malaria parasites in a thick or thin blood film. In non-immune subjects, symptoms may occur when parasitaemia is only at a low level so a careful search for parasites by an experienced microscopist is required, preferably on more than one blood film, before a diagnosis of malaria can be excluded. In contrast, in endemic areas, many asymptomatic subjects have malaria parasitaemia, so detection of parasites in a sick child does not necessarily mean that these are the cause of the child's illness.

Experienced microscopists can detect infections at the level of about 5 parasites per microlitre. Attempts have been made recently to improve the sensitivity of microscopy by using immunofluorescent rather than routine staining techniques but opinion is divided as to whether these new tests, such as the QBC test, are more sensitive than conventional microscopy.[28]

A variety of other diagnostic tests for malaria have been developed recently based upon the detection of parasite antigen, DNA or RNA. None of these tests has yet reached the stage of replacing microscopy as the primary means of diagnosis in an individual patient but some are proving useful in epidemiological surveys and in research situations.

TREATMENT

Antimalarial therapy

Prompt treatment with an appropriate antimalarial drug is an essential first step in the management of a child with malaria but deciding which antimalarial to use can be difficult. Factors that need to be taken into consideration are the species of malaria parasite responsible for the infection, the severity of the infection, the area where the infection was acquired, the pattern of drug resistance in that area and the level of the patient's previous exposure to malaria. Paediatricians who are inexperienced in the management of malaria may consider it prudent to obtain expert advice on the choice of therapy; in the UK this can be obtained from the London or Liverpool School of Tropical Medicine.

Mild infections

Chloroquine can still be recommended as the first line of treatment for non-immune or semi-immune patients infected with *P. vivax, P. malariae* or *P. ovale* (Table 6.2), although chloroquine-resistant *P. vivax* has been detected recently in Papua New Guinea and in Indonesia. Unfortunately, chloroquine-resistant isolates of *P. falciparum* are now widespread in nearly all the areas where this parasite is found so that recommendations for treatments of mild or moderately severe cases of *P. falciparum* infection are more complicated.

The usual treatment for a non-immune child, such as a visitor to an endemic area, with uncomplicated falciparum malaria is oral quinine. However, quinine is unpleasant to take and often induces side-effects, so that ensuring compliance with a full course of treatment can be difficult. If the infection was acquired in Africa, mefloquine or halofantrine are likely to be effective and are more palatable alternatives.

In the malaria-endemic areas of Africa chloroquine is still used widely as a first-line treatment for uncomplicated malaria as it is safe and cheap and generally effective at suppressing symptoms, even if it does not eliminate parasitaemia. However, in several African countries clinical failures with chloroquine are becoming so frequent that a change to an alternative first-line treatment is becoming necessary. Fansidar (pyrimethamine + sulphadoxine) is the generally favoured alternative. In the areas of the Far East where high levels of chloroquine and Fansidar resistance are found, a combination of Fansidar and mefloquine (Fansimef) has been used successfully for many years as the first-line treatment for uncomplicated falciparum malaria in the indigenous population. However, resistance to this drug combination is becoming widespread on the borders of Thailand and in Cambodia where various alternative therapies, including high-dose halofantrine, artemesin derivatives and various drug combinations are being tried.

Severe malaria

Parenteral therapy with quinine is the usual choice of treatment for severe malaria among the population of endemic areas and in visitors to such areas (Table 6.3). However, resistance to quinine is increasing in South-East Asia and so alternative therapies are being investigated. A promising alternative is the artemesin derivative artemether. The efficacy of artemether in severe

Table 6.2   Drugs used in the chemotherapy of uncomplicated malaria in children

Drug	Indications	Dose and duration of treatment	Side-effects	Comments
Quinine	*Plasmodium falciparum* infections in areas of chloroquine resistance	10 mg salt/kg 8-hourly for 7 days	Nausea, vomiting, tinnitus	May be difficult to achieve compliance with full course of treatment. Efficacy can be improved by giving additional tetracycline but this is not advisable in young children
Chloroquine	*P. malariae*, *P. ovale* and *P. vivax* infections. *P. falciparum* infections in semi-immune children from endemic areas with low levels of chloroquine resistance	25 mg base/kg given over 3 days	Nausea and vomiting. Itching in African patients	May suppress symptoms but not parasitaemia in partially resistant infections
Fansidar	Chloroquine-resistant *P. falciparum* infections acquired in West Africa	25 mg/kg sulphadoxine + 1.2 mg/kg pyrimethamine as a single dose	Occasional severe skin reactions and blood dyscrasias	Relatively cheap
Mefloquine	Chloroquine-resistant *P. falciparum* infections	25 mg base/kg as a single dose	Nausea and vomiting. Occasional neuropyschiatric side-effects	Relatively expensive. Should be given with food
Halofantrine	Chloroquine-resistant *P. falciparum* infections	8 mg/kg 6-hourly for 3 doses	Minor gastrointestinal symptoms and occasional pruritus	Relatively expensive. Variable gastrointestinal absorption. Should be given with food. High incidence of recrudescences after a single course of treatment. Thus, some advocate a second dose on day 7

Note: To eradicate *P. vivax* and *P. ovale* infections, which have a secondary liver cycle, primaquine should be given in a dose of 0.25 mg/kg for 14 days. Primaquine may cause severe haemolysis in children with glucose-6-phosphate dehydrogenase deficiency.

malaria has been demonstrated in several uncontrolled studies in South-East Asia and a large comparative trial of quinine and artemether in adults with severe malaria is now underway in Vietnam. Artemether acts more rapidly than chloroquine.[29] Thus, artemether is also being tried in areas of Africa

Table 6.3   Recommended chemotherapy for severe falciparum malaria in children

Drug	Indications	Dose and duration of treatment	Side-effects
Quinine	Severe falciparum malaria in areas with chloroquine resistance	By infusion — loading dose of 20 mg salt/kg over 4 h followed by 10 mg/kg every 8 h until the patient can take oral quinine (10 mg/kg 8-hourly) to complete 7 days of treatment.	Nausea, vomiting, tinnitus, visual disturbances, hypotension, cardiac arrhythmias, hypoglycaemia
		By intramuscular injection — loading dose of 20 mg salt/kg in divided doses followed by 10 mg/kg 8-hourly until oral medication is started.	As above + sterile injection abscesses
		By nasogastric tube — 10 mg salt/kg 8-hourly for 7 days	Less likely to cause cardiovascular toxicity
Artemether	Severe falciparum malaria in an area with some quinine resistance, such as Cambodia	3.3 mg/kg by intramuscular injection followed by 1.6 mg/kg i.m. daily for 4 days	Recrudescences after treatment are frequent

Notes
1. Studies from Africa have shown satisfactory blood quinine levels when a loading dose and 12-hourly treatment regimens have been used.
2. Treatment by nasogastric tube is recommended only in emergency situations when parenteral therapy under supervision is not possible.
3. If patients have already received quinine or mefloquine before presentation, loading doses of quinine should be omitted.
4. Quinidine has been used to treat malaria successfully in adults but there is little experience in the treatment of children with quinidine. It is probably more cardiotoxic than quinine. However, it may be available in hospitals where quinine is not readily accessible. The recommended dose is an initial infusion of 15 mg base/kg given over 4 h followed by 7.5 mg/kg 8-hourly.
5. Artemether is not generally available in Europe or North America.

where parasites are still quinine-sensitive, in an attempt to reduce the high mortality of cerebral malaria.

New antimalarials

In parts of South-East Asia the time is not too far ahead, if it has not arrived already, when cases of malaria will be encountered for which there is no effective antimalarial treatment. Although work is continuing on the development of quinghaosu derivatives and on a new hydroxynapthoquinone antimalarial, atovaquone, development of new antimalarials has not kept pace with the development of resistance in *P. falciparum*, in part because antimalarials are not a commerically attractive proposition for the large pharmaceutical companies. Unless innovative ways can be found of persuading pharmaceutical companies to work on antimalarials, the future of chemotherapy for malaria is bleak.

Supportive treatment

Severe malaria is always a serious condition and, whenever possible, children with severe malaria should be nursed in an intensive care unit with appropriate attention being paid to ventilation and fluid balance. Uncomplicated malaria can be managed on an outpatient basis provided that the paediatrician can be sure that treatment will be given correctly.

Children with malaria often have a high fever which requires treatment with an antipyretic. Anticonvulsants such as paraldehyde or diazepam may be required to control fits which are frequent in children with cerebral malaria. The value of prophylactic phenobarbitone has not been established in children. Children with cerebral malaria are sometimes severely hypoglycaemic so blood sugar levels should be carefully monitored and intravenous glucose given if indicated.

Anaemic patients may require urgent transfusion, as haemoglobin levels can fall suddenly in children with malaria due to rapid clearance of PRBC. In some centres, exchange transfusion is used in the management of patients with high levels of parasitaemia and a poor prognosis[30] but the benefit of exchange transfusion has never been established conclusively in a controlled clinical trial. Patients who develop renal failure may require dialysis.

Because mortality from cerebral malaria remains high despite appropriate antimalarial therapy a variety of additional therapies such as anticoagulants and steroids have been tried without success. Recently it has been reported that an iron chelator desferrioxamine accelerated the rate of recovery of children with cerebral malaria.[31] New knowledge on the pathogenesis of cerebral malaria opens the way to other forms of supportive therapy. Thus, a trial of an anti-TNF monoclonal antibody is being undertaken in The Gambia and treatments that might interfere with cytoadherence of infected RBC to endothelial cells are being investigated.

PREVENTION OF MALARIA

Prevention of malaria can be achieved by destroying the vector; reducing the infectiousness of the vector; preventing contact between humans and the vector; and protecting the host from infection should an infectious bite occur.

Vector control

Elimination of malaria from Europe and the USA was accomplished primarily through vector control, but vector control has generally been much less successful when applied in the tropics. Household spraying is the main method used for destroying adult mosquitoes but the effectiveness of this form of malaria control is now being seriously questioned in many areas because mosquitoes have become resistant to cheap insecticides and/or have changed their behaviour so that they no longer rest in houses. Extensive use of insecticides is expensive and ecologically undesirable.

Molecular biology offers an exciting new approach to vector control. It has been found that some strains of vector mosquitoes are naturally resistant to malaria infection. It is possible that, by genetic engineering techniques, it may be possible to create resistant mosquitoes which are able to displace the susceptible and hence potentially infectious strain.

Reduction of human–vector contact

A substantial measure of protection against mosquito bites can be plished by the use of sensible clothes, mosquito repellents and mosquito coils. When properly used, mosquito nets provide an excellent protection against night-biting mosquitoes but they are of little value if not tucked in carefully or if they are torn. However, treatment of mosquito nets with an insecticide, such as permethrin, increases substantially their protective effect against mosquitoes and other insects, even when they are torn. Trials of insecticide-impregnated bednets carried out in many countries with different patterns of malaria transmission during the past few years have nearly all shown some effect on the vector and/or on the incidence of malaria in the study population.[32] The most dramatic results have come from trials in The Gambia where child mortality has been reduced substantially following the introduction of impregnated bednets combined with chemoprophylaxis.[33]

Chemoprophylaxis

Chemoprophylaxis has transformed the outlook for non-immune visitors to the most malarious areas of the world. Before chemoprophylaxis was used widely, few visitors to West Africa survived for more than a few years. Now malaria deaths among visitors to Africa are rare, although they do still occur. During the past few years the question of who should be given prophylaxis and what prophylactic should be used has been placed on a much sounder scientific basis than in the past.[34] Chemoprophylaxis may not be appropriate for short-term visitors to an area with a low risk of infection, for in these circumstances the risks from the prophylactic drug are likely to exceed those from malaria, or for visitors to areas where parasites are resistant to all conventional prophylactic drugs. However, under most circumstances chemoprophylaxis is appropriate for visitors to endemic areas and should be recommended, the drug chosen being determined by the area to be visited and by any special characteristics of the visitors (Table 6.4).

Table 6.4 Drugs used most widely in the chemoprophylaxis of malaria

Drug	Indications	Contraindications	Prophylactice dose	Side-effects	Comments
Chloroquine	Protection against *Plasmodium vivax*. Protection against *P. falciparum* in areas of low-level chloroquine resistance		5 mg base/kg once per week	Nausea and vomiting. Pruritus in Africans. Retinal damage after large doses (>5kg)	Usually taken with proguanil
Proguanil	Protection against *P. falciparum* in areas of low-level drug resistance	Previous severe mouth ulcers	<2 years 50 mg/day 2–10 yrs 100 mg/day >10 years 200 mg/day	Mouth ulcers	Usually given with chloroquine
Mefloquine	Protection against chloroquine-resistant *P. falciparum*	Children <8 years. Neurological or psychiatric illness. Therapy with cardioactive drugs	15–19 kg 62.5 mg weekly 20–30 kg 125 mg weekly 31–45 kg 187.5 mg weekly	Nausea and vomiting. Bad dreams	Shown to be more effective than chloroquine + proguanil in Africa
Maloprim	Protection against *P. falciparum* in areas of low drug resistance	Infants <3 months	<1 year $\frac{1}{4}$ tablet. (pyrimethamine 3.2 mg; dapsone 25 mg) weekly 1–10 years $\frac{1}{2}$ tablet weekly	Rare blood dyscrasias	Not used widely but still effective in tropical Africa
Doxycycline	Protection against chloroquine- resistant *P. falciparum*	Children <8 years	2 mg/kg daily	Nausea and vomiting. Photosensitive rashes	Only recommended for short courses

Notes

1. Insufficient antimalarials are secreted in breast milk to provide protection, so infants require prophylaxis.
2. Although mefloquine is not recommended by the manufacturers for prophylaxis in children < 8 years there are no indications of enhanced toxicity in children.
3. Fansidar is no longer recommended for prophylaxis because of an unacceptably high level of serious side-effects.
4. When no suitable prophylactic regimen can be recommended, travellers may be advised to take with them halofantrine for use as an emergency treatment when skilled medical help is not available.

Whether chemoprophylaxis should ever be given to the resident population of malaria-endemic areas is controversial. It is generally recommended that chemoprophylaxis should be given to pregnant women, especially primigravidae, resident in malaria-endemic areas because of their increased susceptibility to malaria. Generally chemoprophylaxis has not been recommended for young children permanently resident in an endemic area, except for those with sickle cell disease or for those who are on immunosuppressive drugs, because of fears that chemoprophylaxis will impair their development of natural immunity and accelerate the spread of drug-resistant parasites. However, recent studies the The Gambia have shown that, in an area where drug resistance is not yet a major problem, chemoprophylaxis targeted to children under the age of 5 years was very effective at reducing child mortality and did not lead to either a significant impairment of immunity or to accelerated drug resistance.[35]

Vaccination

The quest for a malaria vaccine has proved to be more difficult than was anticipated 10 years ago when new immunological and molecular biological techniques were first applied to the study of malaria. However, there are strong grounds for believing that development of a malaria vaccine is possible. The ability of a vaccine comprising irradiated sporozoites to give protection against a challenge infection in volunteers, first reported in 1973,[36] has recently been confirmed. Unfortunately, for logistic reasons, an irradiated sporozoite vaccine is not a practical possibility. During the past 10 years susbtantial progress has been made towards the development of vaccines that will induce immune responses against pre-erythrocytic, erythrocytic or the sexual stages of P. falciparum (Fig. 6.1) and trials of all three types of vaccine have been undertaken in humans or are about to start.

Pre-erythrocytic stage vaccines

Unfortunately, subunit pre-erythrocytic vaccines have not been as effective as irradiated sporozoites. Most pre-erythrocytic vaccines studied so far have been based on a sequence of amino acids (NANP) which are repeated many times in the circumsporozoite protein which is present in large amounts on the surface of sporozoites. Various vaccine constructs and adjuvants have been tried. Although several of these vaccines have induced good antibody responses in volunteers, few immunized volunteers have been protected when challenged with infected mosquitoes. Three trials of NANP vaccines in malaria-endemic areas were unsuccessful.[37] Thus, it is likely that these vaccines do not induce the right kind of immunity and attempts to develop more effective pre-erythrocytic stage vaccines, in particular those that induce cytotoxic T-cell responses to liver stage antigens, are continuing.

BLOOD-STAGE VACCINES

In general, the severity of malaria is related to the level of peripheral blood parasitaemia, so that a blood-stage vaccine that could suppress parasitaemia without being able to prevent infection might still provide substantial protection against disease. This appears to be the case for the malaria vaccine SPf 66 which reduced levels of parasitaemia in volunteers without preventing infection.[38] This vaccine, developed in Colombia, consists of three peptides derived from blood-stage antigens which are linked by the NANP repeat of the circumsporozoite protein and then polymerized to form a large immunogenic molecule. Several large trials of this vaccine have been undertaken in South America with reported vaccine efficacy against *P. falciparum* infection of about 50%. These early findings were controversial because of problems with the trial designs[39] but it has been reported that a more recent randomized double-blind trial undertaken in Colombia again showed about 50% protection aginst falciparum malaria. Spf 66 is now undergoing trial in an area of Tanzania where the level of malaria transmission is much higher than in South America. Other blood stage vaccines are reaching the point of phase I–II trials.

Transmission-blocking vaccines

Transmission-blocking vaccines represent a novel approach to vaccine design because they do not protect the vaccinated subject from infection but prevent him or her from spreading the parasite to others. However, because transmission of malaria is usually focal, once all members of a community have been vaccinated then each will achieve a susbtantial degree of protection against infection. A vaccine based on a 25 kD ookinete antigen, expressed by the parasite only in the mosquito, has been developed and shown to be very effective at inducing transmission-blocking antibodies in experimental animals.[40] This vaccine is about to start clinical trials.

Combined control strategies

It is unlikely that any of the first generation of malaria vaccines will be fully protective. Similarly, other established malaria control measures such as insecticide-treated bednets and chemoprophylaxis are only partially effective. Thus, the most promising approach to improving the present malaria situation is the judicious use of combinations of control measures in a way best suited to meet local circumstances.

KEY POINTS FOR CLINICAL PRACTICE

- Malaria must be considered as a possible diagnosis in any febrile child who has recently visited a malaria-endemic area and cerebral malaria must be considered as a possible diagnosis in any such child who has an acute illness with neurological signs or symptoms.

- Low levels of malaria parasitaemia can cause symptoms in non-immune subjects so careful examination of a thick blood film, preferably on more than one occasion, is required before a diagnosis of malaria can be excluded.
- If expert advice on treatment is not available oral quinine is the first choice of treatment for uncomplicated cases of falciparum malaria and parenteral quinine for severe falciparum malaria. Chloroquine should be used for children with *P. malariae, P. ovale* or *P. vivax* infections.

REFERENCES

1 Stürchler D. How much malaria is there world wide? Parasitol Today 1989; 5: 39–40
2 Bate CAW, Taverne J, Roman E, Moreno C, Playfair JHL. TNF induction by malaria exoantigens depends on phospholipid. Immunology 1991; 75: 129–135
3 Schofield L, Hackett F. Signal transduction in host cells by a glycosylphosphatidylinositol toxin of malaria parasites. J Exp Med 1993; 177: 145–153
4 Karunaweera ND, Grau GE, Gamage P, Carter R, Mendis KN. Dynamics of fever and serum TNF levels are closely associated during clinical paroxysms in *Plasmodium vivax* malaria. Proc Natl Acad Sci USA 1992; 89: 3200–3203
5 Kwiatkowski D, Molyneux ME, Stephens S et al. Tumour necrosis factor mediates fever in cerebral malaria. Q J Med 1993: 86: 91–98
6 Sherman IW, Crandall I, Smith H. Membrane proteins involved in the adherence of *Plasmodium falciparum*-infected erythrocytes to the endothelium. Biol Cell 1992; 74: 161–178
7 Howard R, Handunnetti S, Hasler T et al. Surface molecules on *Plasmodium falciparum*-infected erythrocytes involved in adherence. Am J Trop Med Hyg 1990; 43: 15–29
8 Roberts DJ, Craig AC, Berendt AR et al. Rapid switching to multiple antigenic and adhesive phenotypes in malaria. Nature 1992; 357: 689–692
9 Treutiger C-J, Hedlund I, Helmby H et al. Rosette formation in *Plasmodium falciparum* isolates and anti-rosette activity of sera from Gambians with cerebral or uncomplicated malaria. Am J Trop Med Hyg 1992; 46: 503:510
10 Udomsangpetch R, Todd J, Carlson J, Greenwood BM. Effects of HbA and S and ABO antigens on *P. falciparum* rosettes. Am J Trop Med Hyg 1993; 48: 149–153
11 Kwiatkowski D, Hill AVS, Sambou I et al. TNF concentration in fatal cerebral, non-fatal cerebral and uncomplicated *Plasmodium falciparum* malaria. Lancet 1990; 336: 1201–1204
12 Grau GE, Taylor TE, Molyneux ME et al. Tumour necrosis factor and disease severity in children with falciparum malaria. N Engl J Med 1989; 320: 1586–1591
13 Berendt AR, Simmons DL, Tansey J, Newbold CI, Marsh K. Intercellular adhesion molecule-1 is an endothelial cell adhesion receptor for *Plasmodium falciparum*. Nature 1989; 341: 57–59
14 Clark IA, Rockett KA, Cowden WB. Proposed link between cytokines, nitric oxide and human cerebral malaria. Parasitol Today 1991; 7: 205–207
15 Phillips RE, Pasvol G. Anaemia of *Plasmodium falciparum* malaria. Clin Haematol 1992; 5: 315–330
16 Abdalla S, Weatherall DJ, Wickramasinghe SN, Hughes M. The anaemia of *P. falciparum* malaria. Br J Haematol 1980; 46: 171–183
17 Cohen S, McGregor IA, Carrington S. Gamma-globulin and acquired immunity to human malaria. Nature 1961; 192: 733–737
18 Riley EM, Allen SJ, Wheeler JG et al. Naturally acquired cellular and humoral immune responses to the major merozoite surface protein (PfMSP1) of *Plasmodium falciparum* are associated with reduced malaria morbidity. Parasitol Immunol 1992; 14: 321–337
19 Riley EM, Greenwood BM. Measuring cellular immune responses to malaria antigens in endemic populations: epidemiological, parasitological and physiological factors which influence *in vitro* assays. Immunol Lett 1990; 25: 221–229

20 Hill AVS, Elvin J, Willis A et al. Molecular analysis of the association of HLA-B53 and resistance to severe malaria. Nature 1992; 360: 434–439

21 Greenwood B, Marsh K, Snow R. Why do some African children develop severe malaria? Parasitol Today 1991; 7: 277–281

22 Hill AVS, Allsopp CEM, Kwiatkowski D et al. Common West African HLA antigens are associated with protection from severe malaria. Nature 1991; 352: 595–600

23 World Health Organization. Severe and complicated malaria. Trans R Soc Trop Med Hyg 1990; 84 (suppl 2): 1–65

24 Molyneux ME, Taylor TE, Wirima JJ, Borgstein J. Clinical features and prognostic indicators in paediatric cerebral malaria: a study of 131 comatose Malawian children. Q J Med 1989; 71: 441–459

25 Newton CRJC, Kirkham FJ, Winstanley PA et al. Intracranial pressure in African children with cerebral malaria. Lancet 1991; 337: 573–576

26 Brewster DR, Kwiatkowski D, White NJ. Neurological sequelae of cerebral malaria in children. Lancet 1990; 336: 1039–1043

27 Bethell D, Waller D, Dung NM et al. A prospective study of severe malaria in Vietnamese children. In: Tharavanij S, Fungladda W, Khusmith S, Pruekwatana O (eds) Abstracts of the XIIIth International Congress for Tropical Medicine and Malaria, Mahidol University, Bangkok Vol 2. 1992: p. 69

28 Anonymous. QBC in malaria diagnosis. Lancet 1992; 339: 1022–1023

29 White NJ, Waller D, Crawley J et al. Comparison of artemether and chloroquine for severe malaria in Gambian children. Lancet 1992; 339: 317–321

30 Anonymous. Exchange transfusion in falciparum malaria. Lancet 1990; i: 324–325

31 Gordeuk V, Thuma P, Brittenham G et al. Effect of iron chelation therapy on recovery from deep coma in children with cerebral malaria. N Engl J Med 1992; 327: 1473–1477

32 Bernejo A, Veeken H. Insecticide-impregnated bednets for malaria control: a review of the field trials. Bull WHO 1992; 70: 293–296

33 Alonso PL, Lindsay SW, Armstrong JRM et al. The effect of insecticide-treated bednets on mortality of Gambian children. Lancet 1991; 337: 1499–1502

34 Steffen R, Behrens RH. Traveller's malaria. Parasitol Today 1992; 8: 61–66

35 Greenwood BM, Greenwood AM, Bradley AK et al. Comparison of two strategies for control of malaria within a primary health care programme in The Gambia. Lancet 1988; i: 1121–1127

36 Clyde DF, Most H, McCarthy VC, Vanderberg JP. Immunization of man against sporozoite-induced falciparum malaria. Am J Med Sci 1973; 266: 169–177

37 Ballou WR, Hoffman SL, Sherwood JA et al. Safety and efficacy of a recombinant DNA *Plasmodium falciparum* sporozoite vaccine. Lancet 1987; i: 1277–1281

38 Patarroyo ME, Amador R, Clavijo P et al. A synthetic vaccine protects humans against challenge with asexual blood stages of *Plasmodium falciparum* malaria. Nature 1988; 332: 158–161

39 Targett GAT. SPf66, a candidate synthetic malaria vaccine: immunogenicity versus protection. Parasitol Today 1992; 8: 354–355

40 Carter R, Kumar N, Quakyi IA et al. Immunity to sexual stages of malaria parasites. Prog Allergy 1988; 41: 193–214

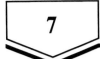

7

Molecular pathophysiology of bacterial meningitis

X. Sáez-Llorens   G. H. McCracken Jr

With the advent of antimicrobial therapy, bacterial meningitis has changed from a disease with an almost universally fatal outcome to one in which most patients now survive. Development of extraordinarily active antibiotics and advanced intensive care technology have been associated with a further, albeit slight, improvement in outcome from this disease. Case-fatality and especially case-morbidity rates remain, however, unacceptably high.[1] At the present time, it is widely believed that for us to improve substantially outcome from meningitis, new treatment modalities based on a better understanding of basic disease mechanisms must be implemented.[2]

Extensive clinical and experimental data generated in recent years have revealed that live meningeal pathogens are not by themselves responsible for the harmful effects on the central nervous system.[3-7] Indeed, clinical expression of meningitis arises largely from the host response to the inciting organism in the subarachnoid space. It is the intensity and duration of this inflammatory reaction that ultimately determines the severity and outcome from this disease. Increasing knowledge of the complex interaction between bacterial offenders and the host mechanisms triggered to eliminate them promises to bring new therapeutic horizons to minimize brain tissue damage.[3,4]

In this review we will briefly describe current concepts of the evolving pathophysiologic events that follow the initial mucosal colonization, local invasion, blood stream survival and meningeal invasion of bacteria and highlight the clinical and therapeutic implications of these processes.

PATHOGENESIS

Host exposure to a meningeal pathogen through colonization of the nasopharyngeal mucosal epithelium is an initial step for development of bacterial meningitis. To attach and invade this mucosa successfully, the organism must first adhere to epithelial cells by means of specific binding receptors located on both bacterial and mucosal surfaces, evade secretory immunoglobulin A challenge through the release of bacterial proteases, avoid the ciliary clearance mechanisms of the nasopharyngeal mucosa, and subsequently traverse the basolateral side of this epithelium.[3,4,8] Although this sequence of events might apply to most neurotropic bacteria, the specific patterns of invasion across the nasopharynx are thought to be different for the various meningeal pathogens. In addition, it is believed that a concurrent viral infection of the upper respiratory tract can facilitate the invasion of the blood from colonizing mucosal sites.[3,4]

Once bacteria gain access to the intravascular compartment, they must overcome additional host defenses for survival. The capsular polysaccharide of most meningeal pathogens confers the ability to avoid the initial alternative complement pathway that does not require specific antibody for activation. Because presence of neutralizing antibodies to capsular antigens that promote opsonization and eradication of the bacteria in the blood stream is age-related, infants and young children are more likely to develop meningitis once bacteria enter the vascular space.[1,3]

Finally, depending on the concentration and peristence of organisms in the blood, central nervous system invasion can occur. The exact mechanisms by which these pathogens penetrate the blood–brain barrier and enter the cerebrospinal fluid are unknown, but specific surface bacterial components and binding receptors on endothelial cells of meningeal capillary vessels and choroid plexus epithelium are likely to be involved.[4] Because of insufficient humoral factors (e.g. antibody, complement) and phagocytic activity in cerebrospinal fluid (CSF), bacteria reaching the subarachnoid space multiply rapidly and liberate active cell wall or membrane-associated products (endotoxin, teichoic acid, peptidoglycans).[3,4] Following these initial complex steps, the pathophysiologic events of meningeal inflammation result in clinical manisfestations of central nervous system infection.

PATHOPHYSIOLOGY

The pathophysiologic events leading to meningeal inflammation, cerebral edema, alterations in CSF hydrodynamics and brain damage commence as a result of release of bacterial products within the subrachnoid space. These products stimulate macrophage-equivalent brain cells (e.g. astrocytes, microglia) and cerebral capillary endothelium to produce potent proinflammatory cytokines, notably tumor necrosis factor-alpha (TNF-α) and interleukin-1 (IL-1).[5,9,10] Initial parenteral antimicrobial therapy can, by provoking an accelerated bacterial destruction, increase the amount of bacterial products in CSF, thereby inducing a transient amplification of the meningeal inflammatory cascade in some patients.[11–16]

These two polypeptide mediators, TNF-α and IL-1, activate surrounding cells to liberate a still-increasing number of inflammatory susbstances (e.g. IL-6, IL-8, phospholipaspe A$_2$, platelet-activating factor, arachidonic acid metabolites, granulocyte-macrophage colony-stimulating factor, macrophage-derived proteins, etc.).[3,4] These host hormones, acting separately or in concert, promote alterations of brain capillary endothelium that lead to disruption of the blood–brain barrier. These changes comprise expression of adhesion-promoting receptors (i.e. immunoglobulin, integrin and the selectin families of receptors) and their complementary ligands on leukocytes and endothelial cells, activation of complement and coagulation pathways, increased blood–brain barrier permeability and passage of plasma components from the vascular compartment into the CSF.[3,4,17]

Once large numbers of neutrophils migrate into the CSF they are stimulated by the same locally produced cytokines to degranulate and release oxygen radicals and other proteolytic substances. These toxic products induce cytotoxic changes in cerebral tissue and, along with serum proteins and other plasma components, increase CSF viscosity and interfere with resorption of this fluid at the arachidonic villi.[3,4,18] The interaction of all these pathophysiologic events can eventually lead to cerebral edema, increased intracranial pressure, loss of cerebrovascular autoregulation, diminished cerebral blood flow and ultimately to an irreversible focal or diffuse brain damage in some patients (Fig 7.1).[3,4,19,20]

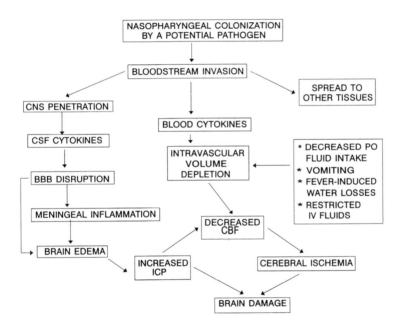

Fig. 7.1 Pathophysiologic events during bacterial meningitis. CNS = Central nervous system; CSF = cerebrospinal fluid; BBB = blood–brain barrier; ICP = intracranial pressure; CBF = cerebral blood flow; PO = per os.

CLINICAL EXPRESSION OF PATHOPHYSIOLOGIC EVENTS IN MENINGITIS

The sequence of events that occur during the course of bacterial meningitis have important clinical consequences in the affected patient (Table 7.1).

Table 7.1 Clinical findings related to pathophysiology

Pathophysiologic event	Clinical findings
Bacteremia	Hypotension or shock, petechiae, disseminated intravascular coagulation, septic arthritis, pneumonia, facial cellulitis, fever, chills
Meningeal inflammation	Fever, meningeal signs, cranial nerve palsies, subdural effusions, early seizures
Cerebral edema, increased intracranial pressure, reduced cerebral blood flow	Lethargy, confusion, headache, focal neurologic findings, bulging fontanelle, herniation of brain structures, coma

Increasing knowledge of these molecular steps within the meningeal inflammatory cascade has fostered promising therapeutic approaches to optimize outcome from disease. For a better general perspective of recent research on meningitis, we will describe, in a sequential fashion, the clinical aspects of the events mentioned earlier and discuss potential therapeutic interventions directed at modulating each of them.

Blood stream bacterial invasion

A variety of clinical findings associated with the presence of meningeal pathogens within the intravascular space can occur either before or during central nervous system bacterial invasion. Cutaneous manifestations such as purpura and petechiae, although most commonly seen with meningococcal disease, can on rare occasions be observed in patients with meningitis caused by any of the bacterial pathogens.[1] Unpublished data of ours indicate that purpuric lesions are seen in 4% of children with meningitis due to *Haemophilus influenzae*. The presence of rapidly progressing purpuric lesions accompanied by hypothermia, disseminated intravascular coagulation and shock, however, is usually associated with infections caused by *Neisseria meningitidis*. Although at the present time it is unknown why some patients with meningococcal disease have a rather benign course whereas others develop a fulminant, rapidly fatal illness, it appears that an overwhelming cytokine-induced host inflammatory response to large endotoxin concentrations in plasma contributes to the severity of disease.[10] Interestingly, patients with terminal complement deficiencies, although more susceptible to meningococcal infections, are less likely to develop fulminant disease than patients with an intact complement system.[1] Accordingly, host factors reacting to the presence of meningococcal endotoxin rather than direct effects of the bacterium itself are likely to be responsible for the severity of this disease.

Besides invading the central nervous system, bacterial agents present in the blood can also migrate to other tissues and cause focal infections such as periorbital or buccal cellulitis, suppurative arthritis and pneumonia. Because these conditions can occur either before or after development of clinical signs of meningitis, a lumbar puncture should be considered part of the initial work-up of many of these patients.

Therapeutic implications

It is reasonable to assume that early administration of appropiate parenteral antimicrobial therapy before a significant bacterial inoculum is reached in the CSF can reduce the clinical expression of bacterial meningitis and prevent the development of complications. Nevertheless, it is important to realize that administration of antibiotics could initially result in worsening of the patient's clinical condition as a result of release of proinflammatory cytokines within the vascular and subarachnoid compartments.[1,16]

Although no prospective clinical studies have evaluated the role of anti-inflammatory therapy given before parenteral antibiotic administration in preventing vascular manifestations associated with bacteremia, it is possible that pharmacologic modulation of cytokine production in the systemic circulation can attenuate these potential complications during the early phases of meningitis. Interestingly, a recent retrospective review suggested that steroid therapy when given before or concomitantly with antibiotic treatment to infants and children with pneumococcal meningitis was associated with a significant reduction in cardiovascular instability, presumably related to administration of the first parenteral antibiotic dose compared with results in patients given placebo.[19] Studies addressing this issue are urgently needed.

Meningeal inflammation

Inflammation of meninges and other nervous tissue structures occurs as a result of passage from the circulation to the CSF of a large number of polymorphonuclear leukocytes resulting from cytokine-induced disruption of the blood–brain barrier. Accumulation of a significant inflammatory mass contributes to development of cytotoxic, interstitial and vasogenic cerebral edema and to complications generated by increased intracranial pressure and reduced cerebral vascular blood flow.[18,20,21] High concentrations of protein and white blood cells in the CSF can also contribute to stagnation of CSF circulation.

Subarachnoid space inflammation is clinically characterized by the presence of meningeal signs and by the early apppearance of focal neurological findings. In many patients in whom a second CSF sample is obtained 12–24 h after the initial specimen, there is an increased pleocytosis.[1,7] Although this phenomenon can be presumably explained by the fact that some patients are diagnosed during an early phase of meningitis when leukocytes are initiating their CSF penetration, there is now strong evidence indicating that the initial antimicrobial therapy, by provoking a rapid bacterial killing and a subsequent explosive release of cell wall products from lysed organisms into the CSF, is largely responsible for this event in those patients.[3,4]

Therapeutic implications

To diminish central nervous tissue inflammation, potential therapeutic agents must interfere with either production of cytokines or with leukocyte-endothelium interaction induced by proinflammatory mediators. Although steroids are the only drugs that have been evaluated in clinical trials, there are other potential therapeutic approaches being tested in experimental animals that might be useful in the near future. It is important to emphasize, however, that for newer agents to be effective in diminishing meningeal inflammation and blood–brain barrier disruption, they should be administered before or simultaneously with the first parenteral dose of an appropriate antibiotic.[12] In addition, we believe that the choice of an antimicrobial agent is critical because significant reduction in the blood–brain barrier permeability as a result of anti-inflammatory therapy is associated with diminished CSF antibiotic concentrations as well.

In all recent experimental and clinical studies of meningitis, dexamethasone given before or concomitantly with third-generation cephalosporins (i.e. ceftriaxone or cefotaxime) has been associated with significant modulation of meningeal inflammation.[6,7,12,19,22-25] When dexamethasone is given at various times after antibiotic therapy, either slight or no reductions of CSF inflammation have been observed in animals.[6,12,19,26] These modulatory effects are in accord with in vitro experiments, in which production of cytokines is inhibited when macrophages or astrocytes are exposed to dexamethasone before their contact with bacterial endotoxin.[27,28]

Pentoxifylline, a phosphodiesterase inhibitor, affects functional properties of polymorphonuclear leukocytes once they are activated by endotoxin or cytokines. In vitro experiments have shown that pentoxifylline decreases the adherence of leukocytes to endothelial cells, reduces generation of superoxide and other toxic oxygen radicals and attenuates the release of proteolytic substances contained within neutrophil granules.[29] In addition, pentoxifylline has been shown to suppress TNF production by endotoxin-stimulated mononuclear cells.[27] Experiments in animals have demonstrated significant reductions in meningeal inflammation and in blood–brain barrier permeability when high doses or continuous intravenous infusions of pentoxifylline are given either before or shortly after intracisternal inoculation of *Haemophilus influenzae* type b organisms or their purified endotoxin.[23,30] Additional studies examining the potential efficacy and safety of pentoxifylline or its derivatives in meningitis models are needed before exploring its clinical applicability.

Another promising therapeutic approach is the administration of monoclonal antibodies directed against adhesion-promoting glycoproteins located on either endothelial or polymorphonuclear cells. To date, only specific antibodies reacting with the β_2 integrin family of leukocyte receptors (i.e. anti-CD18 monoclonal antibodies) have been tested in animals.[24,31] Intravenous administration of these antibodies to rabbits with meningitis induced by live bacteria, endotoxin, pneumococcal cell wall fragments or cytokines significantly reduced the severity of the meningeal inflammatory process and disruption of the blood–brain barrier.[24,31] In addition, a significant attenuation of brain edema was observed in anti-CD18 antibody-treated rabbits, especially when these antibodies were given in combination with dexamethasone.[24] Safety issues related to their administration in humans must be evaluated before these agents can be tested in clinical trials of bacterial meningitis.

Brain edema and increased intracranial pressure

Depending on the magnitude and duration of pathophysiologic changes and the timing of therapeutic interventions, meningeal inflammation is usually associated with varying degrees of cerebral edema and with increased intracranial pressure. Vasogenic edema is primarily a consequence of increased permeability of the blood–brain barrier to the influx of plasma components into the CSF. Cytotoxic cerebral edema results from swelling of the cellular elements of the brain caused by toxic products released by bacteria or degranulated neutrophils. Interstitial edema occurs secondary to obstruction of normal CSF outflow with a subsequent dilation of ventricles or obvious hydrocephalus.

Development of brain edema is a major determinant leading to increased intracranial pressure.[20,21] Transient or sustained increases in cerebral blood flow also can result in increased intracranial pressure, which can have detrimental consequences.[19,32] Intracranial pressures below 60 mm of water for newborns, 80–90 mm of water for infants and young children and 120–150 mm of water for older patients are considered normal.[33] Significant increases in these intracranial pressures can result in life-threatening consequences, especially in children and adults in whom the rigid confines of their skull and spine can lead to cerebral herniation. By contrast, infants and young children by virtue of their open fontanelles and cranial sutures often can tolerate high intracranial pressures without developing herniation of vital cerebral structures.

Therapeutic implications

Several therapeutic approaches are claimed to reduce cerebral edema and increased intracranial pressure. Because high fever augments cerebral blood flow to meet the increased brain's metabolic demands, antipyretic measures are usually implemented. In patients with severe meningitis, hyperventilation, by decreasing $PaCo_2$, produces cerebral vasoconstriction and as a consequence decreases the intracranial pressure by reducing cerebral blood volume.[34] The $PaCo_2$ should be maintained, however, between 25 and 30 mmHg because levels below 20 mmHg can result in cerebral ischemia. Hyperosmolar agents such as mannitol decrease intracranial pressure by decreasing cerebral edema. Mannitol remains almost exclusively in the intravascular space, making this compartment hyperosmolar. The result is movement of water from brain tissue and surrounding extracellular space into the intravascular space.[20] Its effect, however, is transient, lasting approximately 2–4 h.

Nonsteroidal anti-inflammatory drugs, which interfere with the conversion of arachidonic acid to prostaglandins, have been tested in experimental animal models. Indomethacin has been shown to reduce brain edema but not meningeal inflammation and intracranial pressure.[35] Recent evidence indicates that prostaglandins, by acting in a negative feedback manner, are important modulators of TNF and IL-1 production.[3,4] Thus, selective inhibition of the cyclooxygenase metabolic pathway may paradoxically be more detrimental than beneficial.

In several experimental meningitis studies, corticosteroids have been effective in reducing brain edema and intracranial pressure and in enhancing CSF resorption.[15,20,24,36] These beneficial effects appear to be more pronounced with dexamethasone than with methylprednisolone therapy. Additionally, dexamethasone has been shown to reduce significantly antibiotic-induced increases of brain water content and CSF pressure in animals treated with ceftriaxone.[22] The effects of dexamethasone in reducing increased CSF pressure have been confirmed in a recent clinical pediatric trial.[7] In this study, infants and children receiving the first dose of dexamethasone 15–20 min before the first dose of cefotaxime had a lower CSF pressure at 12 and 24 h after enrolment compared with patients who received placebo and cefotaxime. Indeed, placebo recipients had an even higher intracranial pressure at 12 h than that recorded on admission.

Finally, administration of agents directed against endothelium–leukocyte interactions (i.e. pentoxifylline, antiadhesion antibodies), by attenuating the blood–brain barrier disruption and thereby modulating vasogenic, cytotoxic and interstitial edema, could lower intracranial pressure that results from meningeal inflammation. As suggested in one experimental study, it is possible that combined therapy with one of these promising agents and a corticosteroid could be associated with greater reductions than those occurring after either drug given alone.[24]

Cerebral blood flow impairment

In experimental meningitis, cerebral blood flow increases initially followed by diminished flow as inflammation worsens.[4] The initial increased flow is probably related to the generation of oxygen intermediates or cytokine-induced vasoactive substances in the microvasculature, whereas later decreases occur as a result of steady increases in intracranial pressure.[20,37] If these pathophysiologic events are not promptly modulated, loss of cerebrovascular autoregulation ensues and cerebral blood flow becomes mainly dependent on the mean arterial systemic blood pressure.[4] These events have important clinical implications, since inadvertent increases in mean arterial pressure directly increase cerebral blood flow and raise intracranial pressure, whereas decreases in mean arterial pressure can result in diminished cerebral blood flow and reductions in oxygen and glucose delivery to the brain.

Besides cerebral perfusion pressure, other factors such as tissue metabolic demand and blood oxygen and carbon dioxide concentrations can affect cerebral blood flow. Clinical data indicate that reduction of cerebral perfusion pressure below a certain threshold (i.e. < 30–40 mmHg) is associated with death or major neurologic sequelae in children with intracranial infections.[7,32,34] Accordingly, maintenance of mean arterial blood pressure within normal ranges is crucial for achieving optimal cerebral perfusion pressure and for avoiding brain ischemia and progressive cerebral anaerobic metabolism.

Therapeutic implications

Therapeutic modalities designed to reduce brain water content and intracranial pressure are also theoretically effective in improving cerebral perfusion pressure. In a recent prospective study, dexamethasone therapy was associated with increases in estimated cerebral perfusion pressure compared with decreased perfusion pressure in placebo recipients at 12 h after start of therapy.[7] It is likely that therapeutic agents directed to block leukocyte-endothelium interactions will also improve blood flow to cerebral tissue.

It is currently recommended that patients with bacterial meningitis be treated with restriction of intravenous fluids to prevent or ameliorate the syndrome of inappropiate secretion of antidiuretic hormone.[1] A recent clinical study, however, has challenged this traditional dogma.[38] Serum arginine vasopressin was measured on admission and after 24 h of therapy in 13 children with bacterial meningitis. The patients were prospectively randomized to receive either a conventional fluid restriction regimen (60 ml/kg per day) or a maintenance plus deficit replacement regimen (150 ml/kg per day). Serum arginine vasopressin was elevated in both groups at the start of treatment, but 24 h later remained significantly higher in those treated with fluid restriction compared with values in the group given fluids in a liberal fashion.[38] These results suggest that the elevated concentrations of serum arginine vasopressin were an indicator of intravascular volume depletion rather than inappropriate secretion of the hormone. This intravascular volume depletion was probably a result of a decreased fluid intake, vomiting, fever-induced water losses, and of hypotension induced by release of cytokines in the systemic circulation that may occur in children with bacterial meningitis. Accordingly, it is likely that elevated serum arginine vasopressin may be an appropriate physiologic response to intravascular volume depletion in many patients with bacterial meningitis.

Additional evidence supporting these findings comes from an experimental animal model of pneumococcal meningitis.[39] In this recent study, animals receiving a small intravenous fluid regimen (50 ml/kg per day) had a lower mean arterial blood pressure, lower cerebral blood flow, and higher CSF lactate concentrations 16 h after intracisternal inoculation of bacteria compared with animals given a high fluid regimen (150 ml/kg per day).[39] Moreover, larger differences in these systemic and cerebral hemodynamic variables between these two regimens were observed in the first 4–6 h after antibiotic administration. Thus, intravascular volume status appears to be a critical variable in determining outcome from disease. A large clinical trial evaluating different fluid regimens in bacterial meningitis seems justified.

Outcome from pathophysiologic events during bacterial meningitis

The most common sequelae of bacterial meningitis that have been detected in prospective studies include cranial nerve palsies, hemi- or quadriparesis, muscular hypertonia, ataxia, permanent seizure disorders, hearing impairment, cortical blindness, and obstructive hydrocephalus.[1] In addition, infants and children who recover from bacterial meningitis are thought to experience behavioral problems, language disorders (usually related to hearing deficits), and lower intelligence when compared with control children or their healthy siblings. Some of these adverse residual events, however, resolve partially (hearing impairment) or completely (ataxia) with time.

Neurologic sequelae are believed to be a result of brain ischemia and sustained hypoxia of vital cerebral areas and compression of cranial and spinal nerves by the thick inflammatory exudate. The mechanisms responsible for hearing impairment are unknown but presumably involve bacterial products, cytokines and leukocytes in the auditory canal and cochlear aqueduct.[40,41]

Most recent prospective clinical trials performed in infants and children with bacterial meningitis have shown a beneficial effect of dexamethasone therapy on reducing the incidence of hearing impairment or neurologic deficits or both in different populations, especially when dexamethasone was administered before initiation of parenteral antimicrobial therapy (Table 7.2).[6,7,25] The beneficial effect of dexamethasone therapy, however, did not attain statistical significance in some trials because the number of patients studied was too small to achieve statistical power. However, in one study when cefuroxime therapy was used and when a population with a high rate of sequelae was studied, the power was sufficient to attain statistically significant differences in outcome (Table 7.2)

Based on the sequence of pathophysiologic events discussed earlier, late administration of dexamethasone or other anti-inflammatory agents is not expected to result in beneficial effects on long-term outcome from bacterial meningitis. Because most of the patients enrolled in these studies have had

Table 7.2   Children with audiologic and/or neurologic sequelae after receiving early therapy with dexamethasone. Results of recent double-blind, placebo-controlled trials

Place of study	Timing of steroid	Antibiotic employed	Dexamethasone S/TP (%)*	Placebo S/TP (%)*	P value	Reference
Dallas, USA	+ 2–3[†]	Cefuroxime	3/43 (7)	11/38 (29)	0.021	6
		Ceftriaxone	3/49 (6)	9/46 (20)	0.065	6
USA (Multicenter)	+ 2 h	Ceftriaxone	6/68 (8.8)	10/74 (14)	0.434	26
Costa Rica	– 15–20 m[‡]	Cefotaxime	7/51 (14.0)	18/48 (38.0)	0.007	7
Switzerland	– 10 m	Ceftriaxone	3/60 (5.0)	9/55 (16)	0.066[§]	25

* Number of patients with any sequelae/total number of patients, expressed as a percentage.
[†]Average hours after first dose of antibiotic.
[‡]Average minutes before first dose of antibiotic.
[§]When studies using ceftriaxone are combined and assessed by meta-analysis, the incidence of any sequelae in the dexamethasone-treated patients was 6.8% (12 of 177) compared with 15.4% (27 of 175) in placebo recipients (odds ratio: 2.3, 95% confidence interval: 1.2–4.4)

meningitis caused by *H. influenzae* type b, it remains unclear, albeit pathophysiologically plausible, whether patients with pneumococcal meningitis benefit from steroid therapy. A retrospective analysis of such patients provided evidence that dexamethasone therapy was effective in reducing the incidence of neurologic and audiologic sequelae.[19] In addition, because of their usual uneventful clinical course, children with meningococcal meningitis (without systemic vascular manisfestations) seldom develop major sequelae and therefore thousands of patients would need to be studied to detect potential improvements in outcome from steroid therapy.

Better understanding of molecular events that occur in meningitis has provided the basis for a number of new approaches to treatment. Some examples are shown in Table 7.3

Table 7.3   Potential therapeutic modalities directed to various pathophysiologic targets in bacterial meningitis

Pathophysiologic target	Therapeutic modality
Bacterial products in CSF	Endotoxin-neutralizing agents. Drugs to block the activity of bacterial products on their specific receptors
CSF production of cytokines	Steroids, pentoxifylline
Cytokine-induced abnormalities	Steroids, pentoxifylline, cytokine antagonists, antileukocyte adhesion agents
Neutrophil-induced cytotoxicity	Pentoxifylline, oxygen radical scavengers

CSF = Cerebrospinal fluid.

KEY POINTS FOR CLINICAL PRACTICE

- Increased knowledge of the molecular events that occur following invasion of the vascular compartment by meningeal pathogens and after these bacterial agents penetrate into the subarachnoid space has provided the basis for new treatment modalities in addition to conventional antibacterial approaches.

- Experimental and clinical trials have demonstrated that adjunctive dexamethasone therapy reduces production of cytokines in the CSF, modulates meningeal inflammatory indices, and improves outcome from disease.

- It is expected that novel therapeutic agents directed to early sequential steps within the inflammatory cascade (e.g. anticytokine drugs, antileukocyte adhesion agents), especially when used in a timely fashion (prior to antibiotics), will be associated with further improvements in outcome from meningitis.

- Additionally, we believe that the traditional concept of restricting fluids in most patients with bacterial meningitis because of potential development of the inappropriate secretion of antidiuretic hormone syndrome requires re-examination.

REFERENCES

1 Feigin RD, McCracken GH, Klein JO. Diagnosis and management of meningitis. Pediatr Infect Dis J 1992; 11: 785–814

2 Sande MA, Tauber MG, Scheld WM, McCracken GH Jr. Pathophysiology of bacterial meningitis: summary of the workshop. Pediatr Infect Dis J 1989; 8: 929–933

3 Sáez-Llorens X, Ramilo O, Mustafa M, Mertsola J, McCracken GH Jr. Molecular pathophysiology of bacterial meningitis: current concepts and therapeutic implications. J Pediatr 1990; 116: 671–684

4 Quagliarello V, Scheld WM. Bacterial meningitis: pathogenesis, pathophysiology, and progress. N Engl J Med 1992; 327: 864–872

5 Ramilo O, Sáez-Llorens X, Mertsola J et al. Tumor necrosis factor alpha and interleukin-1 beta initiate meningeal inflammation. J Exp Med 1990; 172: 497–507

6 Lebel MH, Freij BJ, Syrogiannopoulos GA et al. Dexamethasone therapy for bacterial meningitis: results of two double-blind, placebo-controlled trials. N Engl J Med 1988; 318: 964–971

7 Odio CM, Faingezicht I, Paris M et al. The beneficial effects of early administration in infants and children with bacterial meningitis. N Engl J Med 1991; 324: 1525–1531

8 Stephens DS, Farley MM. Pathogenic events during infection of the human nasopharynx with Neisseria meningitidis and Haemophilus influenzae. Rev Infect Dis 1991; 13: 22–33

9 Saukkonen K, Sande S, Cioffee C et al. The role of cytokines in the generation of inflammation and tissue damage in experimental Gram-positive meningitis. J Exp Med 1990; 171: 439–448

10 Waage A, Halstensen A, Shalaby R, Brandtzaeg P, Kierulf P, Espevik T. Local production of tumor necrosis factor alpha, interleukin-1, and interleukin-6 in meningococcal meningitis: relation to the inflammatory response. J Exp Med 1989; 170: 1859–67

11 Mertsola J, Ramilo O, Mustafa M, Sáez-Llorens X, Hansen EJ, McCracken GH Jr. Release of endotoxin after antibiotic treatment of Gram-negative bacterial meningitis. Pediatr Infect Dis J 1989; 8: 904–906

12 Mustafa M, Ramilo O, Mertsola J et al. Modulation of inflammation and cachectin activity in relation to treatment of experimental Haemophilus influenzae type b meningitis. J Infect Dis 1989; 160: 818–825

13 Fischer H, Tomasz A. Production and release of peptidoglycan and wall teichoic acid polymers in pneumococci treated with betalactam antibiotics. J Bacteriol 1984; 157: 507–513

14 Tuomanen E, Liu H, Hengstler B, Zak O, Tomasz A. The induction of meningeal inflammation by components of the pneumococcal cell wall. J Infect Dis 1985; 152: 859–868

15 Tauber MG, Schibl AM, Hackbarth CJ, Larrick JW, Sande MA. Antibiotic therapy, endotoxin concentrations in spinal fluid, and brain edema in experimental *Escherichia coli* meningitis. J Infect Dis 1987; 156: 456–462

16 Arditi M, Albes L, Yogev R. Cerebrospinal fluid endotoxin levels in children with *H. influenzae* meningitis before and after administration of intravenous ceftriaxone. J Infect Dis 1989; 160: 1005–1011

17 Springer TA. Adhesion receptors of the immune system. Nature 1990; 346: 425–434

18 Tauber MG, Borschberg V, Sande M. Influence of granulocytes on brain edema, intracranial pressure, and cerebrospinal fluid concentrations of lactate and protein in experimental meningitis. J Infect Dis 1988; 157: 456–464

19 Kennedy WA, Hoyt MJ, McCracken GH Jr. The role of corticosteroid therapy in children with pneumococcal meningitis. Am J Dis Child 1991; 145: 1374–1378

20 Niemöller UM, Tauber MG. Brain edema and increased intracranial pressure in the pathophysiology of bacterial meningitis. Eur J Clin Microbiol Infect Dis 1989; 8: 109–117

21 Fishman RA. Brain edema. N Engl J Med 1975; 293: 706–711

22 Syrogiannopoulos G, Olsen KD, Reisch JS, McCracken, GH Jr. Dexamethasone in the treatment of experimental *Haemophilus influenzae* type b meningitis. J Infect Dis 1987; 155: 213–219

23 Sáez-Llorens X, Ramilo O, Mustafa M et al. Pentoxifylline modulates meningeal inflammation in experimental bacterial meningitis. Antimicrob Agents Chemother 1990; 34: 837–843

24 Sáez-Llorens X, Jafari HS, Severien C et al. Enhanced attenuation of meningeal inflammation and brain edema by concomitant administration of anti-CD18 monoclonal antibodies and dexamethasone in experimental *Haemophilus* meningitis. J Clin Invest 1991; 88: 2003–2011

25 Schaad UB, Lips U, Gnehm HP, Blumberg A, Wedgwood J and the Meningitis Study Group. Dexamethasone therapy for bacterial meningitis: the Swiss experience. 32nd Interscience conference on antimicrobial agents and chemotherapy; Anaheim, California, October 11–14, 1992 (abstract no. 71). Lancet 1993 (in press)

26 Wald E and the US meningitis study group. Dexamethasone for children with bacterial meningitis. In: Program and abstracts of 32nd Interscience conference on antimicrobial agents and chemotherapy; Anaheim, California, October 11–14, 1992 (abstract no. 73) (Submitted)

27 Han J, Thompson P, Beutler B. Dexamethasone and pentoxifylline inhibit endotoxin-induced cachectin/tumor necrosis factor synthesis at separate points in the signaling pathway. J Exp Med 1990; 172: 391–394

28 Velasco S, Tarlow M, Olsen K, Shay JW, McCracken GH Jr, Nisen PD. Temperature-dependent modulation of lipopolysaccharide-induced interleukin-1 and tumor necrosis factor expression in cultured human astroglial cells by dexamethasone and indomethacin. J Clin Invest 1991; 87: 1674–1680

29 Sullivan GW, Carper HT, Novick WJ, Mandell GL. Inhibition of the inflammatory action of interleukin-1 and tumor necrosis factor alpha on neutrophil function by pentoxifylline. Infect Immun 1988; 56: 1722–1729

30 Sable CA, Aubin MA, Scheld WM. Pentoxifylline effect on *Haemophilus influenzae* type b induced alteration in blood–brain barrier permeability in experimental meningitis. In: Program and abstracts of the 31st Interscience conference on antimicrobial agents and chemotherapy; Chicago, September 29–October 2, 1991 (abstract no. 252) (Submitted)

31 Tuomanen E, Saukkonen K, Sande S, Cioffe C, Wright SD. Reduction of inflammation, tissue damage, and mortality in bacterial meningitis in rabbits treated with monoclonal antibodies against adhesion-promoting receptors of leukocytes. J Exp Med 1989; 170: 959–969

32 McMenamin JB, Volpe JJ. Bacterial meningitis in infancy: effects on intracranial pressure and cerebral blood flow velocity. Neurolog 1984; 34: 500–504

33 Mins RA, Engleman HM, Stirling H. Cerebrospinal fluid pressure in pyogenic meningitis. Arch Dis Child 1989; 64: 814–820

34 Goiten KJ, Tamir I. Cerebral perfusion pressure in central nervous system infections of infancy and childhood. J Pediatr 1983; 103: 40–43

35 Tureen JM, Tauber MG, Sande MA. Effect of indomethacin on the pathophysiology of experimental meningitis in rabbits. J Infect Dis 1991; 163: 647–649

36 Scheld WM, Ducey RC, Winn HR, Welsch JE, Jane JA, Sande MA. Cerebrospinal fluid outflow resistance in rabbits with experimental meningitis: alterations with penicillin and methylprednisolone. J Clin Invest 1980; 66: 243–253

37 Pfistes MW, Koedel V, Maberi RL et al. Microvascular changes during the early phase of experimental bacterial meningitis. J Cereb Blood Flow Metab 1990; 10: 914–922

38 Powell KR, Sugarman LI, Eskenazi AE et al. Normalization of plasma arginine vasopresin concentrations when children with meningitis are given maintenance plus replacement fluid therapy. J Pediatr 1990; 117: 515–522

39 Tureen JM, Tauber MG, Sande MA. Effect of hydration status on cerebral blood flow and cerebrospinal fluid lactic acidosis in rabbits with experimental meningitis. J Clin Invest 1992; 89: 947–953

40 Tarlow MJ, Comis SD, Osborne MP. Endotoxin induced damage to the cochlea in guinea pigs. Arch Dis Child 1991; 66: 181–184

41 Kaplan SL, Hawkins EP, Kline MW, Patrick GS, Mason EO. Invasion of the inner ear by *Haemophilus influenzae* type b meningitis. J Infect Dis 1989; 159: 923–930

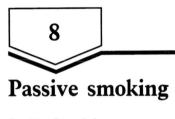

8

Passive smoking

J. M. Couriel

Until the early 1980s, inhaling other people's cigarette smoke was considered a nuisance rather than a health hazard. However, in the last decade, reports from five expert committees have concluded that there is convincing evidence that inhaling the cigarette smoke of smokers can harm the health of non-smokers.[1] Although the risks of such passive smoking are smaller than those of active smoking, they are none the less important. For example, non-smoking adults who inhale the cigarette smoke of others for many years have a risk of developing lung cancer that is 10–30% higher than that of non-smokers who are not regularly exposed to tobacco smoke.[1,2]

Recently there has been increasing interest in the effects of passive smoking on the health of children.[3,4] Children are particularly vulnerable as their respiratory system is structurally and immunologically immature and is developing rapidly. As children spend much of their early life in the presence of their parents, those whose parents smoke will have prolonged and close exposure to environmental tobacco smoke. In the UK, 3.7 million children under the age of 10 live with at least one adult who smokes: in 20% of homes only the mother smokes, in 16% the father smokes, and in a further 13% of homes both parents smoke.[5] Thus, half of the children in this country are exposed to the potential hazards of passive smoking.

The composition and measurement of environmental tobacco smoke

Tobacco smoke in the environment is from two sources. Mainstream smoke is the complex aerosol of over 3500 chemicals that is inhaled by the smoker, filtered by the lungs and exhaled. Sidestream smoke enters the environment directly from the burning tip of a cigarette and accounts for 85% of environmental tobacco smoke. Both types contain gaseous and particulate toxins including carbon monoxide, ammonia, formaldehyde, nicotine and hydrogen cyanide, and over 40 carcinogens includings benzo(a)pyrene, benzene and dimethlynitrosamine. Many constituents are in higher concentrations in sidestream than in mainstream smoke. The amounts of these toxins an individual inhales passively depends on the type and number of cigarettes smoked, the proximity to the smoker, and the size and the ventilation of the room.[1,2]

How can we quantify the 'dose' of environmental tobacco smoke that passive smokers have inhaled? Early studies of passive smoking in childhood relied on a history of whether one or both parents smoked, and in some studies, of the number of cigarettes they consumed daily. Recent studies have quantified exposure by measuring levels of a biochemical marker of tobacco smoke. Cotinine, the prinicipal metabolite of nicotine, is the most sensitive (97%) and specific (99%) indicator of smoking. It can be measured in serum, saliva and urine, and has a half-life of 18–24 h. The salivary cotinine concentration of schoolchildren correlates strongly with the smoking habits of their parents, and particularly with those of their mothers. Cotinine levels correlate closely with air nicotine levels measured within the home and with the results of questionnaires about household smoking.[3] However, Strachan et al also found significant levels of cotinine in children from non-smoking households.[6] This indicates that children are exposed to tobacco smoke from sources other than their parents, and that simply enquiring about parental smoking will underestimate a child's exposure. Cotinine levels are influenced not only by the numbers of smokers in the household, but also by social class, the type of accommodation, day of the week and season of the year.

Although cotinine measurements provided an objective assessment of recent exposure to environmental tobacco smoke, they do not tell us about the duration of exposure or about the intake of other components of tobacco smoke, which may be of more clinical importance than nicotine. Nevertheless, from the data on cotinine levels in passive and active smokers, Jarvis has estimated that the total nicotine dose received by children whose parents smoke is equivalent to their actively smoking between 60 and 150 cigarettes per year.[3]

There are other difficulties in interpreting and comparing studies of passive smoking in children.[4] Prospective, case-control and cross-sectional study designs have been used. Different, often poorly defined, outcome measures have been employed. The degree to which other variables which influence child health, such as socioeconomic status, maternal age and education, prematurity and family size, have been controlled for, varies greatly. It is difficult to separate the intrauterine effects of maternal smoking from the effects of postnatal passive smoking, because 90% of women who smoke during pregnancy are still smoking 5 years later.[7] Despite these difficulties, an increasingly consistent picture of the effects of parental smoking on the health of children has emerged.

PASSIVE SMOKING AND DEATH IN INFANCY

Over a dozen studies have examined the relationship between maternal smoking and death in infancy.[3,4] There has been particular interest in the association between smoking and the sudden infant death syndrome (SIDS), which accounts for 30–48% of all deaths between the ages of 1 week and 1 year in the UK. All but one of these studies have shown that the risk of death to infants of mothers who smoke is two to three times that of mothers who do not smoke during or after pregnancy.[4]

In a study of over 305 000 infants born in Missouri, Malloy and colleagues explored the association between maternal smoking and the age and cause of 2720 infant deaths.[8] The infant mortality rate for all causes was 12.1 deaths per 1000 live births among infants of smokers compared with 7.6 among infants of non-smokers (mean odds ratio 1.6, 95% confidence interval (CI) 1.5–1.7). After adjustment for confounding variables such as the mother's age, parity, education and marital status, and the child's birth weight, smoking was more strongly asssociated with postneonatal death than with neonatal death. The adjusted odds ratio for smoking was particularly high for deaths from respiratory disease (odds ratio 3.4, 95% CI 2.1–3.5) and SIDS (odds ratio 1.9, 95% CI 1.5–2.4). The authors estimated that if no mother had smoked, then the mortality from all causes would have been reduced by 10%, and deaths from SIDS and respiratory illness by 28% and 46% respectively. They also concluded that respiratory deaths and SIDS may be related to postnatal passive exposure of the infant to cigarette smoke, and not simply to smoking during pregnancy.

Haglund & Cnattingius examined maternal smoking as a risk factor for SIDS in a prospective study of 99% of all births in Sweden over a 3-year period.[9] There were 190 cases of SIDS amongst 260 000 live births (0.7 per 1000), representing 27% of all infant deaths between 1 week and 1 year of age. Maternal smoking was the most important preventable risk factor for SIDS. The authors estimated that if maternal smoking could be eliminated, the number of cases of SIDS would be reduced by 27%, an attributable risk remarkably similar to that from the Missouri study.[8] There was a definite dose effect: women who smoked 1–9 cigarettes a day had a relative risk of SIDS of 1.8 (95% CI 1.2–2.6), and those who smoked 10 or more a day had a risk of SIDS 2.7 times higher than non-smoking mothers (95% CI 1.9–3.9). The increased risk associated with smoking was most evident in infants who died in the first 10 weeks of life. These findings agree with data from a UK multicentre study of 988 infant deaths.[4]

A meticulous case-control study of 128 infants with SIDS in New Zealand identified three avoidable risk factors.[10] These were sleeping prone, bottle-feeding and maternal smoking. Smoking in pregnancy increased the risk of SIDS by 2.7 (95% CI 2.5–5.7). There was a strong dose-response effect, with a fivefold increased risk for mothers smoking more than 20 cigarettes a day before their child's death. The attributable risk associated with smoking was 40%, compared to 54% for sleeping prone and 22% for bottle-feeding. The authors concluded that these three risk factors account for 79% of deaths due to SIDS in New Zealand.

Despite their different designs and populations, these studies show that babies born to mothers who smoke have a higher risk of dying in infancy than infants of non-smoking mothers. This risk persists after controlling for other factors associated with infant mortality and is related to the mother's daily cigarette consumption. The risk from smoking is greatest for deaths from respiratory disease and SIDS, the commonest causes of death in this age group. It is not clear how maternal smoking predisposes to infant death, nor do the data allow us to separate between the effects of antenatal and postnatal exposure. However, they do show that maternal smoking is an important and potentially avoidable risk for death in early childhood. If we apply the Swedish attributable risk estimates to data for England and Wales, where there were 1326 deaths classified as SIDS in 1989, elimination of maternal smoking would result in a reduction of these deaths by 365 each year.[3]

PASSIVE SMOKING AND RESPIRATORY ILLNESS

There have been over 18 studies examining the effects of parental smoking on respiratory illness in children. Most have shown an increased frequency of respiratory symptoms of smokers when compared to the children of non-smokers.[2–4]

Respiratory illness in infancy

Twenty years ago, Harlap & Davies, in a prospective study of 10 672 infants, showed a definite dose-response relationship between maternal smoking and hospital admissions for bronchitis and pneumonia[11] Infants of mothers who smoked had an admission rate that was 28% higher than that of infants of non-smokers. Colley et al in a longitudinal study of 2200 chidlren, showed that the incidence of pneumonia and bronchitis was significantly associated with the parents' smoking habits: if both parents were non-smokers the annual incidence was 7.8%, if one parent smoked it was 11.4%, and if both parents smoked it was 17.6%.[12] As in Harlap & Davies' study, the effect of smoking was independent of birth weight, socioeconomic class and family size. In a cohort of New Zealand children followed from birth, Fergusson and associates showed a dose-related effect of maternal smoking on the incidence of pneumonia, bronchitis and bronchiolitis in infancy.[13] Infants of smoking mothers were twice as likely to see a doctor for respiratory illness as infants of non-smokers. Infants admitted to hospital with bronchiolitis or pneumonia caused by the respiratory syncytial virus are more likely to have mothers who smoke than matched control subjects.[14]

In a recent prospective study of 850 infants, the numbers of episodes of wheezing and non-wheezing lower respiratory illness were significantly increased if the mother smoked.[15] The overall odds ratio was 1.5 if the mother smoked, and 1.8 if she smoked more than 20 cigarettes a day. There were no differences between the infants of mothers who smoked both antenatally and postnatally and those who smoked only after birth: the amount smoked was more important than the timing of exposure. Infants of smoking mothers developed respiratory illness earlier than those of non-smokers. Infants who did not attend day-care nursery were at increased risk from maternal smoking, perhaps because they have more prolonged exposure to maternal smoke. In this study, paternal smoking had no detectable effect.

Taylor & Wadsworth[7] and Evans and Golding[4], in retrospective analyses of data from the British National Child Health and Education Study, have confirmed these findings, but have suggested that smoking during pregnancy is more important than smoking in the postnatal period for lower respiratory disease. By contrast, a large study from Shanghai, where women did not smoke during pregnancy, found that the admission rate for respiratory illness correlated significantly with the daily cigarette consumption of family members.[16] This study is important because it demonstrates that postnatal passive smoking has a definite influence on respiratory illness that cannot be explained by maternal smoking during pregnancy.

The increase in lower respiratory disease in infancy caused by passive smoking may have important implications for when the child grows up. Barker & Osmond, in one of an important series of studies of the relationship between infant and adult disease, has found strong evidence of a direct causal link between acute lower respiratory infection in early childhood and chronic bronchitis in adults.[17] They conclude that lung infection during the period of rapid growth in infancy has deleterious effects on lung function which persist into adult life. They suggest that reducing respiratory infection in infancy may reduce the incidence of chronic bronchitis in the next generation.

Respiratory illness in the older child

The relationship between parental smoking and respiratory symptoms in children over the age of 2 is less clear, and some studies that have shown a definite harmful effect in infancy have found no significant effect in older children. Nevertheless, in a prospective study of 4800 5–11 year-olds there was a significant positive association between the frequency of wheeze, cough and episodes of bronchitis and the number of cigarettes smoked by the parents.[18] For example, the relative risk of having frequent wheeze rose from 1.0 if neither parent smoked to 1.3 if they smoked 10 cigarettes a day, and to 1.6 if they smoked 20 per day. Analysis of data from the Harvard longitudinal study revealed a highly significant dose-response relationship between maternal cigarette consumption and the frequency of eight defined respiratory illnesses or symptoms in 6–9 year-olds.[19] Current maternal smoking increased the frequency of these illnesses by between 20 and 35%. Paternal smoking had a smaller but significant effect. A large survey of 8–19-year-olds showed a positive correlation between parental smoking and frequent coughs in children who had never smoked.[20] Thirty-five per cent of boys under 11 whose parents did not smoke reported frequent coughs; if one parent smoked this increased to 42%, and if both smoked the proportion was 48% ($P<0.0001$). The pattern in girls was similar. Mothers' smoking had more influence than fathers'.

Passive smoking and asthma

The studies described so far have examined the effects of passive smoking in unselected populations of children. Children with a pre-existing chronic lung disorder may be particularly susceptible to the adverse effects of environmental tobacco smoke.

Passive smoking increases the frequency and severity of symptoms in children with asthma. Weitzman et al, in an analysis of data on 4000 children aged 0–5 years, found that maternal smoking of more than 10 cigarettes a day was associated with higher rates of asthma (odds ratio 2.1), an increased likelihood of using asthma medication (odds ratio 4.6), and an earlier onset of asthma (odds ratio 2.6) than observed in the children of non-smoking mothers.[21] Hospital admissions with acute asthma were not significantly increased by maternal smoking. In a study of 9670 British children followed from birth, 18% of children had recurrent wheeze by the age of 10.[22] The incidence of recurrent wheeze was increased by 14% when mothers smoked over four cigarettes a day, and by 49% when mothers smoked 15 or more a day. Gortmaker et al found that maternal smoking increased the prevalence and severity of childhood asthma.[23] The attributable risk associated with maternal smoking was estimated to be between 18 and 34% in this population.

In a series of studies of passive smoking and childhood asthma, Murray & Morrison[24-26] have shown that maternal, but not paternal, smoking increases the frequency and severity of asthma symptoms. When compared to asthmatic children whose mothers did not smoke, the children of smoking mothers had lung function indices that were 13–23% lower, and had a fourfold greater degree of responsiveness to an inhaled histamine challenge, indicating airway narrowing and bronchial hyperreactivity.[24] In these studies, boys, and children with atopic dermatitis were particularly susceptible to the adverse effects of maternal smoking, which increased with the duration of exposure to environmental tobacco smoke and the age of the child.[24-26]

PASSIVE SMOKING AND LUNG FUNCTION

The effects of passive smoking on lung function in children and adolescents have been assessed in over 18 studies.[2-4] Most studies have found a significant association between parental smoking and lung function, but others have not. Overall, data from both cross-sectional and longitudinal studies have shown a dose-related reduction in lung function. Maternal smoking appears to be more important than paternal smoking. Younger children and boys appear to be more adversely affected than older children and girls.

Some of the most convincing evidence that passive smoking has a significant effect on lung function has come from the Harvard longitudinal study of childhood risk factors for the development of adult chronic obstructive airways disease. In a 7-year prospective study of 1156 children and adolescents from this cohort, there was a significant association between maternal smoking and lower forced expiratory volume in 1 second (FEV_1) and forced mid expiratory flow rate, two indices of small airways obstruction. Maternal smoking significantly lowered the expected increase in FEV_1 by 7–10% over this period, even after correction for confounding influences.[27]

Few of the studies on lung function have used objective measures of exposure to environmental tobacco smoke. However, two recent cross-sectional surveys of 5–7-year-old children have shown that spirometric indices of airway function are inversely related to salivary cotinine levels, in a pattern suggesting abnormal function of the small airways.[8,28] The differences in lung function indices between those children with the lowest cotinine levels and those in the top fifth of the study population were small (6–7%). In one of these studies,[6] passive smoking did not increase bronchial hyperreactivity, as assessed by the change in lung function in response to exercise. However, in a more detailed study, Frischer et al studied the relationship between maternal smoking and bronchial hyperreactivity as assessed by a standardized exercise test in 1800 schoolchildren.[29] Current exposure to environmental tobacco smoke was not associated with abnormal bronchial hyper-responsiveness, but the odds of being hyperresponsive to exercise were significantly higher in those children exposed to maternal smoking in their first year of life, particularly if they had asthma or positive skinprick tests. A study of young infants showed that parental smoking and a close family history of asthma contributed to the development of bronchial hyperresponsiveness, even at this early age.[30] This evidence suggests that passive smoking in early life may increase bronchial responsiveness, partic-ularly if there is a personal or family history of atopic disease.

Overall, the data from studies of lung function suggest that prolonged passive smoking in childhood results in a reduction in lung size of less than 5%, an effect that is unlikely to produce a detectable health consequence during childhood. However, this reduction may be of relevance to the development of chronic obstructive airway disease as the level of pulmonary function in early adult life is an important predictor of this disease.

Possible mechanisms of lung damage

We do not know the mechanisms by which passive smoking increases respiratory symptoms and decreases lung function in children. Whether passive smoking has a direct toxic effect on the lung or an indirect influence by increasing the child's susceptibility to infection or to the development of atopy is unknown. Parental smoking has been shown to enhance allergic sensitization in infants[31] and schoolchildren[32] with a close family history of atopic disease. In adult smokers, tobacco smoke damages the respiratory cilia and impairs mucociliary transport. Inhalation of tobacco smoke changes the number and function of alveolar macrophages and polymorphs, and causes goblet cell hyperplasia and increased mucus secretion. Changes in antibody and cell-mediated immune responses have also been documented. The relevance of these observations to passive smoking in children is unknown.

EAR, NOSE AND THROAT DISEASE AND PASSIVE SMOKING

Persistent middle ear effusion (glue ear) is the commonest cause of deafness in children and an important cause of delayed language development. Up to 80% of all children will develop an effusion by the age of 5, and 10–20% will have had an effusion in the previous year. Persistent middle ear effusion is the commonest cause for children in the UK to need an operation, and 5–10% of all children have ear, nose and throat surgery for this condition.[33]

Many factors influence the development of persistent middle ear effusion. In a detailed case-control study of the aetiology of persistent middle ear effusion, Black showed that parental smoking significantly increased the risk of undergoing surgery for this condition in 150 children aged between 4 and 9 (mean relative risk 1.64, 95% CI 1.1–2.2).[34] In a population-based study of 700 7-year-old schoolchildren, the overall prevalence of middle ear effusion, as measured by impedance tympanometry, was 9.4%.[33] There was a highly significant trend for more abnormal tympanograms with higher salivary cotinine levels. One-third of effusions in this age group were attributable to passive smoking. Iversen et al found that parental smoking was the only home environmental factor that influenced the prevalence of middle ear effusion.[35] By calculating the attributable risk, they estimated that parental smoking accounted for 15% of effusions in children aged 1–7, and 36% of cases in 6–7-year-olds.

In a longitudinal study of 130 children below the age of 3, the relationship between passive smoking, as assessed by serum cotinine levels, and middle ear effusion, as assessed by pneumatic otoscopy, was studied.[36] Children with high cotinine levels had a 38% higher rate of episodes of otitis media with effusion than children with low levels. The episodes of effusion lasted significantly longer in children with high cotinine levels (28 versus 19 days respectively). After allowance for other variables, 8% of episodes and 18% of days of otitis media with effusion were attributable to passive smoking in this age group.

The mechanism by which passive smoking causes middle ear disease is unclear. Tobacco smoke may have a direct effect on the mucosa of the middle ear causing oedema, abnormal mucociliary clearance, blockage of the Eustachian tube, and impaired ventilation of the middle ear. There may be an indirect effect by adenoidal enlargement, or by increasing infections.

Parental smoking also affects the noses and throats of children.[3] There is a significant association between the frequency of sore throats in children and maternal smoking. There is also a clear dose–effect relationship between habitual snoring in children and parental cigarette consumption, suggesting passive smoking has a chronic effect on the upper airways of children. In a study of the relationship between the number of cigarettes smoked by the parents and a history of adenoidectomy and tonsillectomy, children who had two parents who smoked were almost twice as likely as the children of non-smokers to have had such surgery. As most children have adenotonsillectomy because of recurrent or persistent ear or upper airways symptoms, it has been concluded that passive smoking increases the frequency or severity of these symptoms.

PARENTAL SMOKING AND GROWTH

Infants born to mothers who have smoked during pregnancy are lighter and shorter than infants of non-smoking mothers.[3,4] But does passive smoking also affect postnatal growth? Berkey and colleagues assesssed the association between passive smoking, attained height and height velocity.[37] Children of smoking mothers were shorter than those of non-smoking mothers ($P<0.001$). There was a negative correlation between the attained height and the number of cigarettes the mother smoked daily. The authors made no correction for the parents' heights, the level of smoking during pregnancy or the child's birth weight. The differences in height were small: if the mother smoked 10 or more cigarettes a day, then the mean height of her child was 0.65 cm less than that of a non-smoking mother. Because there were no differences in the height velocities of the two groups, the authors concluded that the differences in attained height were the result of exposure to cigarette smoke in early childhood or in utero.

Rona et al studied children enrolled at birth into the National Study of Health and Growth.[38] The height of the child was significantly associated with the number of cigarettes smoked by the parents, even after allowing for the parents' heights, the child's birth weight, maternal smoking during pregnancy and other factors. The number of cigarettes smoked at home was more strongly related to the height than the number in pregnancy. Father's smoking had a small effect. Children whose parents smoked more than 10 cigarettes a day were on average 0.6 cm shorter than those of non-smoking parents.

These and other[4] studies suggest that children of parents who smoke are slightly shorter than children of non-smokers. It is unclear whether the association is a causal one: social factors associated with adult smoking can also influence growth and development and are difficult to control for in statistical analysis. Whether the effect of passive smoking on height is indirect, for example by increasing respiratory infections in early childhood, or it is a direct toxic effect, is also unclear. Whilst the possible mechanisms are of interest, the magnitude of the effect is of little clinical significance.

OTHER EFFECTS OF PASSIVE SMOKING

Three studies have documented an increase in hospital admissions amongst the children of mothers who smoke. Harlap & Davies calculated a relative risk of admission of 1.2 amongst the infants of mothers who smoked during pregnancy, when compared to non-smoking mothers.[11] Rantakallio recorded a relative risk of 1.35 for hospital admissions amongst 0–5-year-olds whose mothers had smoked during pregnancy.[39] There was a similar relative risk in British 0–5-year-olds from the 1970 birth cohort study.[40] In this study admissions were related to the mothers' smoking habits when the child was 5 and not simply during pregnancy. After adjustment for confounding variables, there was a significant dose-response relationship between the number of cigarettes smoked by the mother and the risk of hospital admission. Using the relative risks from the 1970 birth cohort study, it has been estimated that in England and Wales a minimum of 17 800 children under the age of 5 are admitted to hospital each year as a result of their mothers' smoking.[3]

Smokers' materials are the most frequent cause of fatal house fires, accounting for 39% of all deaths due to ignition in 1990.[3] Some 70–95 children in the UK die each year in house fires, and many more are seriously and permanently damaged.

Evidence is now emerging that prolonged passive smoking during childhood may be important in the development of 'adult' diseases. As discussed previously, passive smoking in childhood may prove to be an important contributory factor to chronic obstructive airways disease in adults. In a case-control study of lung cancer, it was estimated that approximately a sixth of cases of lung cancer in non-smokers can be attributed to high levels of exposure to cigarette smoke during childhood and adolescence.[41] As described in detail elsewhere,[3] the smoking habits of the parents are one of the most important influences on whether their children will themselves become active smokers in adolescence.

CONCLUSIONS

Paediatricians can no longer afford to be complacent about the hazards of passive smoking. Identifying and accepting the problem is important, but it is only the first step. We now need to implement effective strategies to reduce the prevalence of smoking in young people, for these are the parents of tomorrow.[1–3] We need to recognize that despite recent health education campaigns, the prevalence of smoking in teenagers, and particularly in young girls has not reduced in the last decade.[3]

The recent report from the Royal College of Physicians, Smoking and the Young, made many recommendations on how the proportion of young people who smoke could be reduced.[3] These include a ban on all forms of tobacco promotion, an increase in the real price of cigarettes, the introduction of no-smoking policies in schools and public places, and teaching children how to resist the pressures to take up smoking in the first place. Many of these recommendations have already been successfully implemented in parts of this country or abroad. Early studies of improved health education of pregnant women about the hazards of smoking and the setting up of smoking cessation groups in antenatal clinics are promising.[4]

At the very least, paediatricians, and all of those responsible for the health of children, should routinely ask parents about smoking in the home and inform them of the risks to their children that their smoking represents. Given the available evidence, we can tell parents that avoiding smoking during pregnancy and after their child is born offers an opportunity to reduce significantly the risk of illness in their children. Parents who already smoke but wish to give up need to be offered informed guidance and continuing support. This will require liaison between paediatricians, general practitioners and local community services, such as smoking cessation clinics.

The challenge for us is clear. Will paediatricians join with other professionals to reduce the important hazard to the health of children that passive smoking represents?

KEY POINTS IN CLINICAL PRACTICE

- Passive smoking imposes a significant, and potentially avoidable, burden on the health of children.
- Tobacco smoke is the commonest and most important indoor environment pollutant. It contains carcinogens and other toxic chemicals. Children raised in a home where an adult smokes will inhale these toxins throughout childhood and adolescence.
- Maternal smoking during pregnancy and infancy is an important cause of infant death. Over a quarter of sudden infant deaths can be attributed to the mother's smoking. Elimination of maternal smoking would substantially reduce deaths from SIDS and respiratory disease.
- Children of smokers are more likely to be admitted to hospital with respiratory illness in infancy, more likely to suffer from bronchitis, pneumonia and bronchiolitis, and more likely to have recurrent wheeze or cough, than the children of non-smokers.
- The excess respiratory illness caused by passive smoking is most serious in the first 2 years of life. Mother's smoking is more important than father's. The greater the number of cigarettes smoked, the greater the effect on the child.
- Parental smoking significantly increases the frequency and severity of the symptoms of childhood asthma.
- Passive smoking in childhood results in significant changes in lung function, indicating abnormal function of the small airways, and may predispose to chronic respiratory illness in adult life.
- Passive smoking is an important contributor to persistent middle ear effusion, the commonest cause of deafness and the commonest reason for surgery in childhood.
- The hypothesis that there is a causal relationship between passive smoking and these diseases is supported by the consistency of the studies, the

detection of components of tobacco smoke in children, the dose–response relationship between the number of cigarettes smoked and the risk of illness, and by the biological plausibility of such effects. The hypothesis is not weakened by the absence of an understanding of the mechanisms by which tobacco smoke produces these effects: the molecular basis of the link between smoking and lung cancer or atherosclerosis may still be debated, but that there is a causal relationship is now proven.

REFERENCES

1 Wald NW, Booth C, Doll R et al (eds). Passive smoking — a health hazard. London: Imperial Cancer Research Fund and Cancer Research Campaign. 1991
2 Fielding JE, Phenow KJ. Health effects of involuntary smoking. N Engl J Med 1988; 319: 1452–1460
3 Working Party of the Royal College of Physicians. Smoking and the young. London: Royal College of Physicians. 1992
4 Poswillo D, Alberman E, eds. Effects of smoking on the fetus, neonate and child. Oxford: Oxford University Press. 1992
5 Callum C, Johnson K, Killoran A. The smoking epidemic: a manifesto for action in England. London: Health Education Authority. 1992
6 Strachan DP, Jarvis MJ, Feyerabend C. The relationship of salivary cotinine to respiratory symptoms, spirometry and exercise-induced bronchospasm in seven-year old children. Am Rev Respir Dis 1990; 142: 147–151
7 Taylor B, Wadsworth J. Maternal smoking during pregnancy and lower respiratory tract illness in early life. Arch Dis Child 1987; 62: 786–791
8 Malloy MH, Kleinman JC, Land GH, Schramm WF. The association of maternal smoking with age and cause of infant death. Am J Epidemiol 1988; 128: 46–55
9 Haglund B, Cnattingius S. Cigarette smoking as a risk factor for sudden infant death syndrome: a population based study. Am J Public Health 1990; 80: 29–32
10 Mitchell EA, Scragg R, Stewart AW et al. Results from the first year of the New Zealand cot death study. NZ Med J 1991; 104: 71–76
11 Harlap S, Davies AM. Infant admissions to hospital and maternal smoking. Lancet 1974; i: 529–532
12 Colley JRT, Holland WW, Corkhill RT. Influence of passive smoking and parental phlegm on pneumonia and bronchitis in early childhood. Lancet 1974; ii: 1031–1034
13 Fergusson DM, Horwood LJ, Shannon FT. Parental smoking and respiratory illness in infancy. Arch Dis Child 1980; 55: 358–361
14 Pullan CR, Hey EN. Wheezing, asthma, and pulmonary dysfunction 10 years after infection with respiratory syncytial virus in infancy. Br Med J 1982; 284: 1665–1669
15 Wright AL, Holberg C, Martinez FD, Taussig L and Group Health Medical Associates. Relationship of parental smoking to wheezing and non-wheezing lower respiratory tract illnesses in infancy. J Pediatr 1991; 118: 207–214
16 Chen Y, Li W, Yu S. Influence of passive smoking on admissions for respiratory illness in early childhood. Br Med J 1986; 293: 303–306
17 Barker DJP, Osmond C. Childhood respiratory infection and adult chronic bronchitis in England and Wales. Br Med J 1986; 293: 1271–1275
18 Somerville SM, Rona RJ, Chinn S. Passive smoking and respiratory conditions in primary school children. J Epidemiol Community Health 1988; 42: 105–110
19 Ware JH, Dockery DW, Spiro A, Speizer FE, Ferris BG. Passive smoking, gas cooking and respiratory health of children living in six cities. Amer Rev Respir Dis 1984; 129: 366–374
20 Charlton A. Children's coughs related to parental smoking. Br Med J 1984; 288: 1648–1649
21 Weitzman M, Gortmacher SL, Walker DK, Sobol A. Maternal smoking and childhood asthma. Pediatrics 1990; 85: 505–511
22 Neuspiel DR, Rush D, Butler NR, Golding G, Bijur PE, Kurzon M. Parental smoking

and post-infancy wheezing in children: a prospective cohort study. Am J Public Health 1989; 79: 168–171

23 Gortmaker SL, Walker DK, Jacobs FH, Ruch-Ross H. Parental smoking and the risk of childhood asthma. Am J Public Health 1982; 72: 574–579

24 Murray AB, Morrison BJ. The effect of cigarette smoke from the mother on bronchial hyperresponsiveness and severity of symptoms in children with asthma. J Allergy Clin Immunol 1986; 77: 575–581

25 Murray AB, Morrison BJ. Passive smoking by asthmatics: its greater effect on boys than on girls and on older than younger children. Pediatrics 1989; 84: 451–459

26 Murray AB, Morrison BJ. It is children with atopic dermatitis who develop asthma more frequently if the mother smokes. J Allergy Clin Immunol 1990; 86: 732–739

27 Tager IB, Weiss ST, Muno A, Rosner B, Speizer F. Longitudinal study of maternal smoking and pulmonary function in children. N Engl J Med 1983; 309: 699–703

28 Cook DG, Whincup PH, Papacosta O, Strachan DP, Jarvis MJ, Bryant A. Relation of passive smoking as assessed by salivary cotinine concentrations and questionnaire to spirometric indices in children. Thorax 1993; 48: 14–20

29 Frischer T, Kuehr J, Meinert R et al. Maternal smoking in early chidhood: a risk factor for bronchial responsiveness to exercise in primary-school children. J Pediatr 1992; 121: 17–22

30 Young S, le Souef PN, Geelhoed GC et al. The influence of family history of asthma and parental smoking on airway responsiveness in early infancy. N Engl J Med 1991; 324: 1168–1173

31 Arshad SH, Matthews S, Gant C, Hide DW. Effect of allergen avoidance on development of allergic disorders in infancy. Lancet 1992; 339: 1493–1497

32 Ronchetti R, Bonci E, Cutrera G et al. Enhanced allergic sensitisation related to parental smoking. Arch Dis Child 1992; 67: 496–500

33 Strachan DP, Jarvis MJ, Feyerabend C. Passive smoking, salivary cotinine concentrations, and middle ear effusion in 7 year old children. Br Med J 1989; 298: 1549–1552

34 Black N. The aetiology of glue-ear — a case-control study. Int J Pediatr Otorhinolaryngol 1985; 9: 121–133

35 Iversen M, Birch L, Lundquist GR, Elbrond O. Middle ear effusion and the indoor environment. Arch Environ Health 1985; 40: 74–79

36 Etzel RA, Pattishall EN, Haley NJ, Fletcher RH, Henderson FW. Passive smoking and middle ear effusion among children in day care. Pediatrics 1992; 90: 228–232

37 Berkey SC, Ware JH, Speizer FE, Ferris BG. Passive smoking and height growth of preadolescent children. Int J Epidemiol 1984; 13: 454–458

38 Rona RJ, Chinn S, DuVeFlory C. Exposure to cigarette smoking and children's growth. Int J Epidemiol 1985; 14: 402–409

39 Rantakallio P. Relationship of maternal smoking to morbidity and mortality of the child up to the age of five. Acta Paediatr Scand 1978; 67: 621–631

40 Golding J, Haslum M. Hospital admissions. In: Golding J, Butter NR (eds) Birth to five. Oxford: Pergamon Press, 1986 pp. 242–254

41 Janerich DT, Thompson WD, Varela LR et al. Lung cancer and exposure to tobaco smoke in the household. N Engl J Med 1990; 323: 632–636

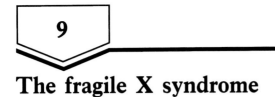

9

The fragile X syndrome

M. C. Hirst   K. E. Davies

The fragile X syndrome is the most common form of inherited mental retardation. Due to rapid progress over the past few years, we now have a basic understanding of the mutation responsible for the syndrome, and can apply this knowledge in its diagnosis and hence its counselling. A gene identified at the fragile X site and mutations within it provide an explanation for the unusual inheritance patterns of the fragile X syndrome and give insights into the puzzling genetics of other common genetic disorders. In this chapter, we summarize the clinical presentation, genetics and diagnosis of the fragile X syndrome and discuss the implications and application of the new molecular tests.

FREQUENCY AND POPULATION GENETICS

The fragile X or Martin–Bell syndrome is the most common single recognized form of inherited mental retardation. It is carried on the X chromosome and thus the syndrome affects more males than females. It is associated with the appearance of a rare folate-dependent fragile site at Xq27.3, visible cytogenetically in metaphase chromosomes from lymphocytes of affected individuals which have been cultured under the appropriate conditions of folate deficiency. It is a common disorder: estimates of its frequency in all human populations range from 0.3 to 1 per 1000 in males and 0.2 to 0.6 per 1000 in females.[1] Up to 50% of all X-linked mental retardation (XLMR) may be attributable to the fragile X syndrome.[2]

THE CLINICAL PHENOTYPE

The fragile X syndrome is characterized clinically by a triad of postpubertal symptoms: moderate mental retardation with an IQ typically in the range 35–50, elongated facies (associated with oedema, tissue thickening and prognathism), with large everted ears, and macro-orchidism.[3] This triad of symptoms is seen in approximately 60% of fragile X males and the variation in their severity is wide, even within families. In males, early symptoms are speech and language delay; hyperactivity with short attention span, poor eye contact, a reluctance to be touched and confused speech. In addition, connective tissue disorders, possibly related to elastin fibre dysmorphism, have been noted. These include joint hyperextensibility, soft velvety skin, puffy eyelids, flat feet and cardiac abnormalities. About 80% of adult patients show mitral valve prolapse. Problems in diagnosis can occur, as 10% of affected males have normal facial features, up to 30% of affected males have no macro-orchidism and 10% present with mental retardation as the only clinical symptom.

Female heterozygotes for the fragile X syndrome are of two types. The first type, daughters of normal transmitting males, almost never show symptoms of the fragile X syndrome and do not express the fragile site cytogenetically. In the second type, granddaughters of normal transmitting males and sisters of affected males, the clinical spectrum is much broader and a large number have no typical features. In those who are cytogenetically positive, over 50% will have some typical features with over 75% showing prominent ears and an extreme shyness. This lack of a distinct heterozygote female phenotype may actually mask the presence of the mutation at a much higher level in the population than has been previously estimated.

Many studies have been carried out of the psychological impairment in fragile X males and carrier females. A high proportion, up to 30%, of fragile X males fulfil the required criteria for classification as autistic, an area of interest which is under continual discussion. Approximately one-third of heterozygous female siblings of affected males are intellectually impaired. Approximately 30% of heterozygotes have been found to exhibit some signs of schizophrenic disorders, and 40% show aspects of affective disorder. Investigations into the structure of the brains in fragile X individuals have recently shown by magnetic resonance scanning that heterozygotes have hypoplasia of the posterior vermis, consistent with developmental and neuropsychiatric disorders.[4]

THE EXPRESSION OF CHROMOSOME FRAGILITY

Fragile sites are detected on human chromosomes microscopically as gaps in one or both chromatids in the metaphase chromosome (Fig. 9.1).[5-7] Their appearance can be induced chemically using suitable biochemical agents. The dicovery that X chromosome fragility was closely associated with mental retardation in some males was pivotal in the recognition of XLMR as an important human disorder. In the case of the fragile X syndrome this is found on the long arm of the X chromosome, at Xq27.3, and is called FRAXA. It is induced under culture conditions of folate deficiency, excess thymidine or in the presence of several chemical additives which disrupt folate metabolism.

The detection of a fragile site at Xq27.3 in mentally retarded male patients has been used as the standard diagnostic test for the fragile X syndrome. Approximately 5% of samples referred for cytogenetic screening because of developmental delay or mental retardation are found to be fragile X-positive.

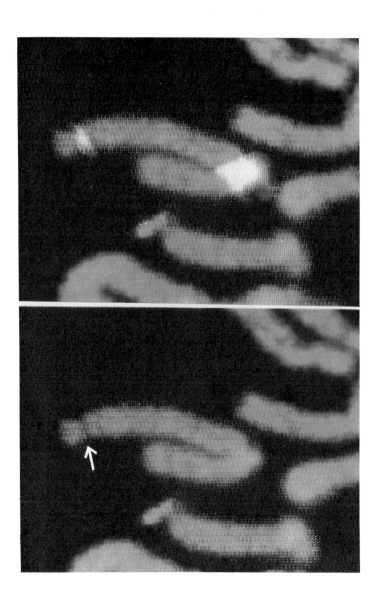

Fig. 9.1 A typical fragile X chromosome seen using fluorescent microscopy. **Left:** the X chromosome, with the region of chromosome fragility clearly visible as a constriction (arrow). **Right:** the localization of an X chromosome centromere probe and the localization of a DNA probe from the FMR-1 region directly over the gap in the metaphase chromosome.

There are, however, several reported cases in which the fragile X site expression and the fragile X syndrome phenotype are dissociated within a sibship. A family segregating for a fragile site in Xq27–q28, but without mental retardation, has also been reported. Affected females generally express the fragile site, but unaffected obligate carrier females (not daughters of normal transmitting males) express the fragile site in less than 50% of cases. The use of cytogenetics for carrier detection has therefore been limited by this.

DNA STUDIES AND THE GENETICS OF FRAGILE X INHERITANCE

Early genetic linkage analysis confirmed that the disease locus mapped to the same region of the X chromosome as the fragile X site (see Fig. 9.1). For an X-linked disorder, the fragile X syndrome is unusual in that transmission of the mutation can occur through apparently normal males. This was first demonstrated using polymorphic DNA markers to study the segregation of the X chromosome in fragile X families. A large collaborative study further revealed that, in addition to the male transmission, there is an imbalance in the penetrance of the phenotype in the different generations of kindreds segregating for the disorder.[8,9] For example, there were fewer than expected affected male sibs of normal transmitting males. The mothers and daughters of normal transmitting males were almost never affected, in contrast to the sisters of affected males, who showed 35% penetrance. The overall penetrance in males was estimated at 79%. The likelihood of developing mental impairment is dependent upon an individual's position in the pedigree. As the mutation progresses through generations, the risk of mental impairment increases. These observations are not consistent with classical X linkage, and are collectively known as the Sherman paradox.

As further new DNA markers became available, their use was developed into a diagnostic strategy based upon genetic linkage analysis. This involved a combination of cytogenetic and extensive family studies. In parallel, these markers were also eventually used to identify the FMR-1 gene, mutations of which give rise to the fragile X syndrome.

THE DISCOVERY OF THE GENE FOR THE FRAGILE X SYNDROME

Intense molecular genetic investigation led to the isolation of the gene responsible for the fragile X syndrome (for review, see Hirst & Davies[10]). Two alterations to this gene occur to give rise to the full clinical phenotype: an amplification of an unusual triplet of DNA and an abnormal methylation of this region leading to the silencing of the FMR-1 gene.

The FMR-1 gene, its structure and expression

The FMR-1 gene is transcribed as a 4.4 kb messenger RNA (mRNA) and is found at high levels in several tissues, including the brain, lung, placenta, kidney and the testes. A second transcript of 1.2 kb in heart tissue has also been described but the relevance of this is as yet unknown. Developmental analysis has shown that FMR-1 is widely expressed during early fetal development. Such early expression suggests that a loss of expression of FMR-1 would have wide-reaching effects. Low levels of expression of the gene in peripheral blood lymphocytes has allowed a study of transcription in fragile X individuals carrying the pre- and full mutation.[11] Such studies have shown that the gene is transcribed in non-penetrant individuals, but is not expressed in affected individuals.

Little is known about the FMR-1 protein, as a comparison of the predicted protein composition and structure with other known proteins identifies only weak similarities. Thus the isolation of the FMR-1 gene represents the identification of a novel gene, perhaps the first in a new family. We await to see how the expression patterns of FMR-1 and its role in cell and tissue functions relate both to mental impairment and to the dysmorphic features with which sufferers of the fragile X syndrome present. The FMR-1 gene is highly conserved in other species (i.e. the DNA sequence of the gene has been maintained through evolution), indicating a conserved cellular function. Thus, further investigations in transgenic animal model systems may well provide critical clues as to its function.

Amplification of a DNA triplet within the FMR-1 gene

The FMR-1 gene has a structure typical of many genes within the human genome. It consists of a series of coding regions, exons, and a transcription control region, or promoter, from which the mRNA production is initiated (Fig. 9.2a). The promoter in the FMR-1 gene is typical of those found in many human housekeeping genes. Such genes are constitutively expressed in most tissues and have promoters which are capable of modification by methylation.

Immediately adjacent to this promoter region, within the first exon of the FMR-1 gene, lies the region of DNA in which the fragile X mutation occurs. The number of CGG repeats on the normal X chromosome varies up to around 50 copies, and these are stably inherited. On the fragile X chromosome, however, the number of repeats increases in a stepwise fashion, eventually leading to the loss of the gene expression.[12-16] The pattern and degree of amplification provide a molecular explanation for the puzzling genetics of the fragile X syndrome and provide a tool for its accurate diagnosis.

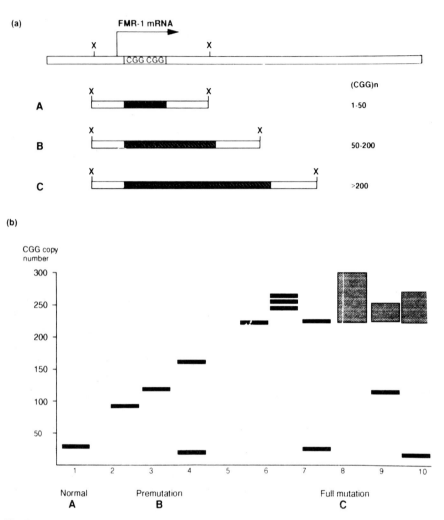

Fig. 9.2   (a) A map of the FMR-1 region and the position of the CGG triplet repeat. The expansion in CGG copy number results in increased-size fragments when analysed with the restriction enzyme X. The fragments shown are the typical CGG copy number in the classifications: A = normals; B = premutations; C = full mutations. (b) The increase in size of the triplet repeat is detected by Southern blot analysis after digestion with a restriction enzyme cutting at site X (for details of which enzymes can be used, see Table 9.2 and text). As the fragment size increases, the migration upon electrophoresis decreases, so larger fragments appear further up the Southern blot. Some typical patterns observed for each mutation class are shown diagrammatically. A1 = Normal; B2,3 = normal transmitting male; B4 = premutation carrier female; C5, 6,8 = full mutation male; C7, 10 = full mutation females; C9 = mosaic male.

Hypermethylation of the FMR-1 gene on the fragile X chromosome

As the CGG array progresses through a fragile X family, the copy number increases until it reaches a critical point; the promoter region undergoes a second change resulting in the silencing of the gene.[17,18] This modification, methylation, appears to mimic the silencing mechanism usually found upon the female inactive chromosome. This process of X-inactivation involves the silencing of gene expression from one of the X chromosomes in females to allow for equal gene dosage between male and females. This silencing is reflected in the methylation of most housekeeping gene promoters on the inactive X chromosome. On the single male X chromosome the promoters are unmethylated. Abnormal methylation is found only in individuals carrying the full mutation. Its presence correlates with the loss of FMR-1 gene expression and cytogenetic fragility.

DIAGNOSTIC APPROACHES

Genotypic profiles of the fragile X chromosome

On the fragile X chromosome, the FMR-1 CGG array can exist in two states dependent upon the CGG copy number.[19,20] This is shown in Figure 9.2 and Table 9.1. Expansion of the CGG repeat can be directly detected by analysis of the size of DNA fragments crossing the mutation region. Individuals carrying a premutation chromosome (e.g. normal transmitting males and their daughters) have a copy number of repeats higher than in the normal population but which is below 200 copies. The repeat number is somatically stable within the individual and the FMR-1 region is non-methylated. It is, however, highly unstable upon transmission from generation to generation, mutating with a frequency of 1 (that is, in 100% of meioses); 95% of the changes result in an increase in the size of the array.

Affected individuals carry a repeat array usually greater than 200 copies, the FMR-1 promoter is hypermethylated and the chromosome exhibits cytogenetic fragility. The mutant allele in these individuals frequently

Table 9.1 The allele states of the FMR-1 gene: CGG expansion length, FMR-1 gene expression, cytogenetic expression of fragility, methylation modification and clinical phenotype

Expansion	Methylation	FMR-1 mRNA	FX expression	Phenotype
<50 CGG	No[*]	Normal	Negative	Normal
50–200	No[†]	Normal	Negative[‡]	Normal
>200	Yes	None	Positive[§]	Affected[**]

[*]The region undergoes normal X inactivation in a female.
[†]Some individuals in this size range have been found to be methylated. In these cases, no FMR-1 mRNA is produced and the individuals are cytogenetically positive and clinically affected.
[‡]16% of females are positive.
[§]All males are cytogenetically positive, but only 77% of females are positive.
[**]Only 50% of females carrying this full mutation are affected.

exhibits somatic variation, often resulting in either multiple fragments or a heterogeneous smear of fragments on Southern blot analysis.

The analysis of fragile X heterozygote females is more complicated. The daughters of normal transmitting males, who are unaffected and cytogenetically negative for fragile X expression, have a mutant allele within the non-penetrant premutation size range. Several patterns for the mutant allele are found in other heterozygotes. Those females with defined fragments of increased size in the non-penetrant range are phenotypically normal. Females where the mutation is visualized as a smear of fragments fall into the classification of both unaffected and affected. Although there are general trends in the relationship in carrier female phenotype to genotype, this area still remains to be clarified. There are several factors which may contribute to this lack of certainty. Firstly, in many cases, the clinical assessment of phenotype in females is incomplete. Secondly, the expression of the carrier phenotype may depend upon the proportion of cells in which the mutant chromosome is the 'active' chromosome, and the distribution of these cells within the body. More detailed psychometric assessment is needed in order to study in further detail the genotype–phenotype relationship.

Strategies for the diagnosis of fragile X syndrome

For diagnostic purposes, molecular changes at the FMR-1 gene can be used as a direct test for the prediction of clinical phenotype. These are particularly important for identifying carrier males and females, which is not possible cytogenetically. Unlike many other human genetic diseases, these tests are unusual in the fact that the interpretation of many of the results is complicated by the very nature of the mutation itself.

Southern blot assays

Southern blot tests utilize several restriction digests and DNA probes. Using restriction enzymes which cut the DNA either side of the CGG expansion region (e.g. at site X on Fig. 9.2a), a fragment of known length is released and

Table 9.2   Diagnostic restriction digest assays for assessing the fragile X mutation

Restriction enzyme	Detects	Confirmed by
EcoRI*	All affected males	
	>90% small mutations	PstI test
PstI†	Size all premutations	Direct PCR
	Normal alleles	Direct PCR
BgIII*	Heterogeneous alleles	
EcoRI + BssHII or EagI*	Methylation status of FMR-1	

*In combination with the DNA probes 0×1.9, pE5.1, Pfxa7 or StB12.3.[10]
†In combination with the probes 0×0.55 or PX6 or Pfxa3.[10]

can be analysed for size by electrophoresis. The choice of enzyme in use depends upon the size of fragment released and the size of amplification present (Table 9.2). Use of the most commonly used enzyme, EcoRI, is shown in Figure 9.3a. This illustrates the detection of the increased fragment in affected males and several carrier individuals. This detects the full mutation in > 99% of cases. Exceptions to this rule have been either mosaic individuals or have a single fragment premutation range which is fully methylated; these can be further investigated with the enzyme PstI, or can be analysed using the polymerase chain reaction (PCR)-based test (see below). This enzyme releases a fragment of smaller size and upon electrophoresis smaller increases in the fragment size are more accurately detected. Thus this serves to size small premutations more accurately. In situations when the full heterogeneous mutation cannot be seen upon EcoRI analysis, the use of the enzyme BgIII is recommended. It serves to compress sufficiently the signal so as to give a detectable signal on a Southern blot. This is particularly useful with the heterogeneous allele in a carrier female wher the smear of fragments above the normal fragment is difficult to resolve as it appears extemely diffuse. This is illustrated in Figure 9.3b. The diffuse heterogeneous mutation is compacted in three females (tracks 2,4 and 6). In this particular family, the heterogeneous fragments in an extreme mosaic male can just be detected (track 1).

PCR-based tests

The development of PCR-based CGG amplification tests has complemented the more time-consuming Southern blot techniques.[21,22] They offer a rapid analytical test, although some problems with detecting full mutations do occur requiring verification of some samples by the Southern blot methods. For the determination of normal and small allele lengths these PCR reactions are the optimum test. A typical result analysing the normal alleles is shown in Figure 9.4a. This clearly illustrates the variation within the population of the length of the CGG.

Polymorphic markers and exclusion mapping

An additional assay can be used to follow the fragile X mutation chromosome; closely linked polymorphic markers. The ones of most use for this type of analysis are the FMR-1 CGG repeat itself and two closely linked polymorphic markers.

The markers named FRAXAC1 and FRAXAC2 flank the CGG region and no genetic recombination has been reported between them.[23] In cases where the mutant haplotype at these loci is known, screening of other individuals can be used to corroborate the direct CGG amplification assays. These markers are useful in exclusion mapping, as shown in Figure 9.4b. The carrier mother has alleles A and C corresponding to her two X chromosomes.

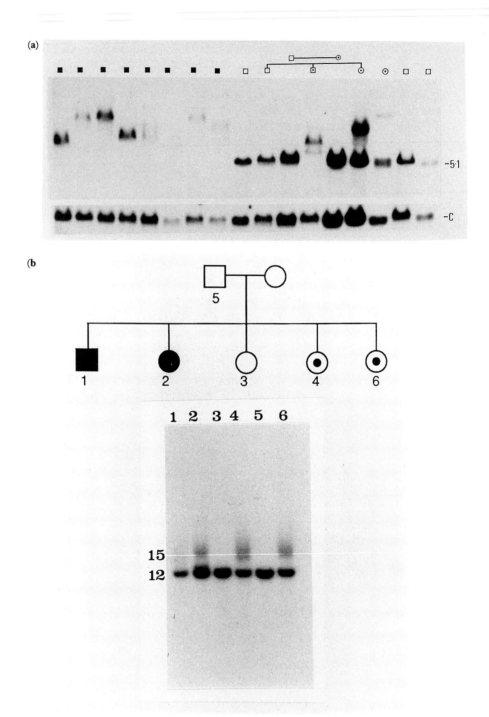

Fig. 9.3 Examples of Southern blot analyses of fragile X individuals showing amplification of the fragile X CGG repeat. □ = Normal male; ○ = normal female; ■ = affected male; ● = affected female. Symbols with central dots represent carrier individuals with no clinical manifestation. (a) Analysis of several individuals and a small family with the enzyme EcoRI and DNA probe 0 × 1.9. The normal fragment is 5.1 kb in size. The lower panel shows the hybridization of a control probe (C) used to demonstrate the loading of DNA in each track. (b) Analysis of a small fragile X family with BglII used to compact the heterogeneous mutation in several females (lanes 2,4,6) and an extreme mosaic male (lane 1).

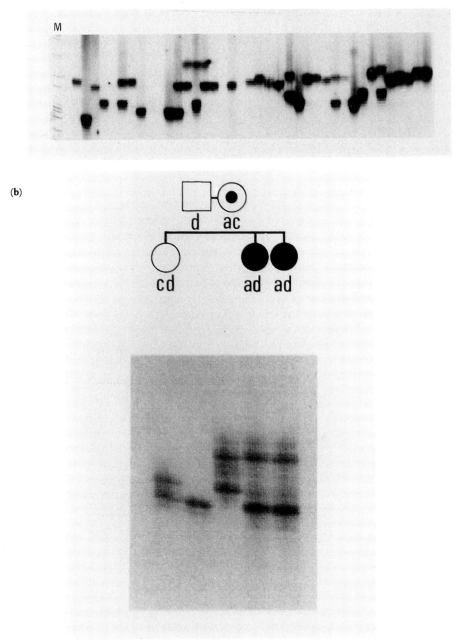

Fig. 9.4   (a) Polymerase chain reaction (PCR) analysis of the normal FMR-1 CGG alleles in 34 individuals ranging in size from 12 to 40 copies. This demonstrates the variation of the CGG length in the population, illustrating its use as a polymorphic marker for genetic analysis. M indicates the marker track used to size these alleles. (b) PCR analysis of the close polymorphic marker FRAXAC1 and its use in excluding the inheritance of the fragile X chromosome. Two affected daughters have inherited the fragile X mutation, which segregates with the A allele from their mother. The normal daughter is confirmed as being a non-carrier as she has inherited her mother's normal C allele.

Her two affected daughters have both inherited her A allele and the D allele from their father. Her other daughter inherits the normal chromosome marked by allele C, and is thus not a carrier for the fragile X syndrome.

As the CGG array itself is a polymorphic marker, normal CGG alleles segregating in a family can also be tracked, allowing the exclusion of the mutation in an individual by demonstrating the inheritance of the normal parental alleles.

The role of cytogenetics

The cytogenetic detection of the fragile X site has played a major role in the detection of the fragile X syndrome over the past years. It is estimated that around 5% of those referred for cytogenetic screening due to significant developmental delay, severe learning difficulties or mental retardation have tested positive. An additional 5% of tested samples carry other constitutional chromosomal abnormalities, indicating that performing a routine chromosome analysis should remain an integral part of the diagnostic procedure for patients demonstrating mental retardation or significant developmental delay due to other causes than the fragile X syndrome.

DNA-based diagnosis will become the primary diagnostic tool in identifying new families as multiple samples can be screened rapidly and cost-effectively. Once a proband is identified, extended family analysis will be carried out solely with DNA tests as these can detect normal transmitting males and their carrier daughters who are cytogenetically negative.

The future of diagnostic tests

DNA screening for the fragile X syndrome is still in a phase of verification. The screening of large cohorts of fragile X patients and families will yield valuable information as to the use of the tests in routine clinical laboratories. Whilst DNA testing will inevitably be more streamlined, the isolation of monoclonal antibodies specific to the FMR-1 protein should lead to the development of further tests.

Prenatal diagnosis

Both in amniocentesis (sampled cells derive from the fetal genitourinary tract) and postnatal diagnoses, the combined analyses of amplification and methylation are readily performed.[24-26] Although the amplification test is accurate, it is important to perform both tests as a small number of several affected males have been found with a premutation-sized amplification.[20] These males are, however, fragile X-positive, and carry a methylated FMR-1 gene. Predicting the phenotype on amplification alone would in these cases have been inaccurate.

In the first trimester, prenatal diagnosis using DNA from chorion villus samples can only be based upon analysing the CGG array amplification at the FMR-1 locus.[24–26] This is because methylation patterns on the X chromosome are not consistently maintained in extraembryonic material. The degree to which we can assay methylation *in utero* still requires further investigation. Patterns of fetal methylation change during development, but are generally not maintained in chorionic material. Thus, until further validation results are known, the interpretation of a premutation in early fetal tissues is still difficult and should be undertaken with care. In the case of chorion villus sampling, further analysis of fetal-derived tissue at a later stage should be considered.

Our ability to perform accurate DNA tests for the fragile X mutation greatly improves the detection of normal carrier males and females. In the case of females carrying the full mutation, however, the tests are of no predictive value as only 50% of females carrying the full mutation will be mentally retarded. For example, the family illustrated in Figure 9.3b has two unaffected carriers and an affected female with indistinguishable mutations. At this moment, we are unable to distinguish those who will be of normal intelligence from those who will be clinically affected.

Mosaicism

The nature of the amplification of the CGG repeat element leads to mosaicism between individual cells. This is normally resolved on Southern blot analysis of a leukocyte sample as a heterogeneous smear of fragments. Individuals have been identified, however, where the mosaicism is between mutation classes, i.e. a sample gives a mixture of pre- and full mutation (see Figs 9.2 and 9.3b). Such mosaics, as expected, express lower levels of the gene and hence less protein.

Consideration must be given to the possibility of the extreme mosaic showing tissue variation throughout the body. This scenario could give rise to individuals who carry a premutation in their leukocytes, carrying the full mutation in the germline. This phenomenon may explain a few cases of clinically affected individuals who, upon DNA analysis of leukocyte DNA, carry a non-methylated premutation. It is possible that such individuals carry the full mutation in a tissue critical for the development of the clinical phenotype.

Fragile X-negative, Martin-Bell phenotype individuals: other mutations in FMR-1

Confirmatory evidence that mutations in the FMR-1 gene are causative of the fragile X syndrome has come from studying individuals with the clinical phenotype of the fragile X syndrome but who are unusual in that they are cytogenetically negative for fragile X site expression. One such fragile X-negative, Martin-Bell phenotype male was found to carry a de novo microdeletion of less than 250 kb across the FMR-1 gene region.[27] He is the first child of non-consanguineous healthy parents with delayed global and speech development, an IQ of 55 and the typical features of the fragile X syndrome. Molecular investigation revealed that the CGG trinucleotide repeat motif and a portion of the FMR-1 gene were deleted. A second similar case has also been described in which the deletion is over 2000 kb of DNA.[28]

A fragile X-negative individual was recently reported carrying a point mutation in the FMR-1 gene which leads to an altered amino acid in the FMR-1 protein.[29] He presented in a family also segregating for X-linked liver glycogenesis, but his additional facial features were typical of the fragile X syndrome. His other features appear to be much more severe than found in the two deletion cases discussed above; a very low IQ (20) and extreme macro-orchidism. Whether this single point mutation is enough to give rise to this severe phenotype, or whether he carries additional alteration elsewhere in the gene, has yet to be determined.

We would predict other individuals will present with the clinical phenotype of the fragile X syndrome, in whom the stepwise amplification of the CGG repeat is absent. Further study of these cases should increase our knowledge of the functions of the FMR-1 gene. Their detection in routine diagnostic assays has yet to be developed effectively, but will rely heavily upon the recognition of the fragile X phenotype in the absence of positive cytogenetic and amplification tests.

Fragile X-positive, CGG amplification-negative families

Cytogenetic analysis for the expression of the fragile X site has been used as the diagnostic criteria in the fragile X syndrome and, by definition, all affected males exhibit the fragile site in their lymphocytes. Several families have been identified who do not have amplification mutations at the FMR-1 locus, but who appear to be cytogenetically positive. Investigation of the site of chromosome fragility in these individuals has led to the identification of two novel fragile sites in Xq27–q28, called FRAXE and FRAXF.[30-32] These sites lie further distal to the FRAXA site, but are impossible to distinguish upon normal cytogenetic investigation. Thus these families have been incorrectly diagnosed as fragile X syndrome.

It is not known whether these sites are causative of the mental retardation in these families, or whether they represent an ascertainment bias for coincidence of fragile X expression and XLMR due to the efficiency of cytogenetic screening. There are many other genes in this region and it will be of great interest to isolate candidate genes in the vicinity of FRAXE and FRAXF.

MODELS FROM OTHER DISEASE GENES

A triplet repeat expansion in the genes for myotonic dystrophy and Kennedy's disease

Amplifications of trinucleotide repeats have also recently been identified at several other loci. In a manner similar to that in fragile X syndrome, the affected status is also associated with an increase in allele length due to the amplification of the repeat array. In the case of Kennedy's disease (X-linked spinal and bulbar muscular atrophy), a CAG trinucleotide in the first exon of the androgen receptor gene has been found to expand in size in affected individuals.[33] The expansion in this gene is small compared to the fragile X syndrome, but this may reflect a functional restraint upon the degree of expansion. As the repeat lies within the protein-coding region of the androgen receptor, a larger expansion might give rise to a non-functional protein, leading to androgen insensitivity and testicular feminization.

In myotonic dystrophy an unstable CTG repeat is present within the 3′ untranslated region of the MT-PK gene, which encodes a putative myotonin protein kinase.[34] Like the fragile X repeat, the allele length increases in subsequent generations, providing a molecular explanation for the clinical feature of anticipation in myotonic dystrophy. The length of expansion is found to correlate with the clinical severity of the disease, with severely affected individuals having alleles with up to 2000 copies of the repeat. In contrast to the fragile X syndrome, in which expansions to the full mutation occur only in the female germline, the molecular expansions in myotonic dystrophy and spinal and bulbar muscular atrophy occur in both the male and female lineages.

PROGRESSION OF THE FRAGILE X MUTATION

The fragile X mutation and the Sherman paradox

In the premutation range, the CGG repeat array is genetically highly unstable, increasing in size from generation to generation.[21] The final expansion to the full mutation depends upon two features: the length of the premutation and the parent from whom the allele is inherited. When inherited from a male, the allele alters in size, occasionally decreasing, but never progresses to a full mutation. This explains why the daughters of normal transmitting males are never clinically affected. In contrast, when inherited from a female, the risk of expansion to a full mutation is purely dependent upon the length of the allele. Detailed analysis of the CGG array demonstrates that, in successive generations descendant from a premutation, it will steadily increase in size, giving a higher probability of progression toward a fully penetrant mutation. Thus the nature of the repeat itself and its expansion provide a molecular explanation for the Sherman paradox, where the penetrance of the disease increases in successive generations.

Timing of the CGG expansion

The FMR-1 CGG array expands progressively, but the exact timing of the expansion is not yet known. It is possible to draw certain conclusions about the timing from several observations. Firstly, mutations found in mosaic individuals are a mixture of the premutation and the full mutation. As we know that most mutations in the CGG array are expansions, it seems unlikely that such individuals started from a full mutation and that a proportion of cells reverted to a premutation size. This suggests that the mutation is inherited as a premutation and expands to the full mutation in early embryogenesis. Mosaics would arise when expansion does not occur early enough in embryogenesis to be present in all progenitor cell lineages. Secondly, the children of the few affected males who have successfully reproduced inherit a premutation-sized allele, suggesting that either the full mutation reverts in spermatogenesis or that a sperm carrying a full mutation is either not viable or not produced.

Postfertilization, expansion occurs very rapidly, as demonstrated by the presence of a heterogeneous full mutation in chorion villus sample material.[24–26] The tissues of an affected fetus show expansion and methylation in all tissues, although the patterns of each are variable between tissues.[35] The stage at which methylation occurs, and whether it plays a role in the normal embryological switching of FMR-1, are unknown.

Population genetics: the pool of predisposed individuals

Segregation studies in fragile X families have suggested an overall carrier rate if 1/800 individuals.[36] As the reproductive fitness of affected hemizygous and heterozygous females is low, and the mutation is constantly being lost from the population, this high frequency requires an explanation. Sherman et al suggested that a high rate of new mutations, in the order of 7.2×10^{-4} in sperm, would account for this high frequency.[8,9] This would suggest that over half of carrier females would be new mutations — something which has not been confirmed with molecular data. As no sporadic cases of the fragile X syndrome have been found carrying the fragile X expansion, the mutation must be being carried through generations by normal transmitting males and normal carrier females. An alternative hypothesis, that unaffected carrier individuals have a selective reproductive advantage, has been suggested.[37] In this case, compensation for the loss of mutant allele in reproductive failure is through a higher reproductive ability of unaffected and mildly affected individuals.

With the isolation of the FMR-1 gene and flanking polymorphic markers, it is now possible to map genetic haplotypes on the fragile X chromosome.

Such studies have revealed linkage disequilibrium around the fragile X mutation.[38] Linkage disequilibrium mapping is based upon the observation that, in close proximity to the mutant gene, chromosomes descended from a common ancestral mutation show a common haplotype reflecting that of the original ancestral chromosome. These observations suggest that most of the fragile X mutations we see today are the result of one or a few founder mutations.

The suggestion that many fragile X chromosomes are line descendants from an ancestral mutation is contradictory to the suggested high mutation needed to explain the high population frequency (see above). To unite these two models, it has been suggested that the pathway of mutation in the fragile X syndrome is a multistep process.[39] The model suggests that alleles of over 50 copies of CGG arise from normal alleles, but these are non-phenotypic and stable for many generations. This longevity would allow the required time for the establisment of an ancestral haplotype, resulting in the observed linkage disequilibrium. The second important aspect of this model is that it is proposed that these larger CGG alleles convert to premutations at a frequency of 1–2% per generation. Once in this state, alleles are highly unstable and progress rapidly to what is seen as full fragile X mutations. This rapid expansion would therefore account for the high mutation rate observed in family studies. Thus it appears that there may be a pool of predisposed individuals from whom the full fragile X mutation is constantly arising.

GENETIC SCREENING AND COUNSELLING

Screening of the general population for a genetic mutation requires due consideration of the problems and benefits of such a test to both society and the individual. Experience from previous screening programmes, for example those with thalassaemia, needs to be taken into account.[40] Amongst these considerations are the reliability and predictive value of the test, the feasibility of carrying out tests, the question as to who has access to the results and the provision of resources to fund such a screening programme. Initial screening programmes could take the form of screening at-risk individuals, such as those with unexplained mental retardation in schools or institutions.

Screening for the fragile X syndrome presents particular problems because of difficulties surrounding the clinical phenotype of heterozygotes and the fact that the predominant phenotype is mental retardation and therefore difficult within society. There are clear advantages to performing a diagnostic test, both to the individual and the relatives. For an affected individual, early diagnosis allows an early intervention and targeting of educational needs, whereas for the family it both reduces the search for a diagnosis and allows informed reproductive choices. Several ethical dilemmas, most prominently in the case of diagnosing carrier males and their daughters, are unique to fragile X syndrome. These individuals will have no medical problems related to the premutation that they carry, but their children or grandchildren will be at risk of carrying a full mutation. Within both the families and the community, identifying such individuals has implications of the problems of third-party discrimination and stigmatization. These risks must be weighed against the right to know held by the individual concerned.

If the fragile X syndrome is indeed an established mutation, as evidence to date from linkage disequilibrium studies suggests, then the frequency of carriers for the predisposing allele within the population may be extremely high. As our understanding of this area progresses, it must be taken into account when screening extended families, where screening for the predisposing haplotype may become feasible.

SUMMARY

The identification of the FMR-1 gene, the CGG amplification events and our subsequent understanding of many of the phenomena of the fragile X syndrome have occurred in a very short space of time. As such, we are very much entering a phase of verification of test procedures and clarification of their interpretation.

KEY POINTS FOR CLINICAL PRACTICE

- The fragile X syndrome is the most common form of XLMR having a phenotype of a large forehead, large ears, long face and macro-orchidism.
- The unusual genetics of the syndrome are explained by a novel form of hereditary DNA mutation leading eventually to the loss of gene expression critical to brain function.
- Accurate and rapid molecular testing is now available to diagnose all carriers and affected individuals of the fragile X syndrome. Genetic counselling and extended family screening are greatly improved.

REFERENCES

1 Webb T. The epidemiology of the fragile X syndrome: In: Davies KE, ed. The Fragile X syndrome. Oxford: Oxford University Press, 1989: 40–45
2 Glass IA. X linked mental retardation. J Med Genet 1991; 28: 361–371
3 Fryns J-P. X-linked mental retardation and the fragile X syndrome: a clinical approach. In: Davies KE, ed. The fragile X syndrome Oxford: Oxford University Press, 1989: 1–39
4 Reiss AL, Freund L, Tseng JE, Joshi PK. Neuroanatomy in fragile X females: the posterior fossa. Am J Hum Genet 1991; 49: 279–288
5 Lubs HA. A marker X chromosome. Am J Hum Genet 1969; 21: 231–244
6 Sutherland GR. Fragile sites on human chromosomes: demonstration of their dependence on the type of tissue culture medium. Science 1977; 197: 256–266
7 Tommerup N. Gytogenetics of the fragile site at Xq27. In Davies KE, ed. The fragile X syndrome. Oxford: Oxford University Press, 1989: 102–135
8 Sherman SL, Morton NE, Jacobs PA, Turner G. The marker (X) syndrome: a cytogenetic and genetic analysis. Ann Hum Genet 1984; 48: 21–37
9 Sherman SL, Jacobs PA, Morton NE et al. Further segregation analysis of the fragile X syndrome with special reference to transmitting males. Hum Genet 1985; 69: 289–299
10 Hirst MC, Davies KE. The fragile X syndrome. Clin Genet 1992; 83: 255–264

11 Pieretti M, Zhang F, Fu Y-H et al. Absence of expression of the FMR-1 gene in fragile X syndrome. Cell 1991; 66: 817–822

12 Verkerk AJMH, Pieretti M, Sutcliffe JS et al. Identification of a gene (FMR-1) containing a CGG repeat coincident with a breakpoint cluster region exhibiting length variation in fragile X syndrome. Cell 1991; 65: 905–914

13 Yu S, Pritchard M, Kremer E et al. Fragile X genotype characterized by an unstable region of DNA. Science 1991; 252: 1179–1181

14 Kremer EJ, Pritchard M, Lynch M et al. Mapping of DNA instability at the fragile X to a trinucleotide repeat sequence p(CCG)n. Science 1991; 252: 1711–1718

15 Nakahori Y, Knight SJL, Holland J et al. Molecular heterogeneity of the fragile X syndrome. Nucleic Acids Res 1991; 19: 4355–4359

16 Oberle I, Rousseau F, Heitz D et al. Instability of a 550bp DNA segment and abnormal methylation in fragile X syndrome. Science 1991; 252: 1097–1102

17 Bell MV, Hirst MC, Nakahori Y et al. Physical mapping across the fragile X: hypermethylation and clinical expression of the fragile X syndrome. Cell 1991; 64: 861–866

18 Vincent A, Heitz D, Petit C et al. Abnormal pattern detected in fragile X patients by pulsed filed gel electrophoresis. Nature 1991; 329: 624–626

19 Hirst MC, Nakahori Y, Knight SJL et al. Genotype prediction in the fragile X syndrome. J Med Genet 1991; 28: 824–829

20 Knight S, Hirst M, Roche A et al. Molecular studies of the fragile X syndrome. Am J Med Genet 1991; 43: 217–223

21 Fu Y-H, Kuhl DPA, Pizzuti A et al. Variation of the CGG repeat at the fragile X site results in genetic instability: resolution of the Sherman paradox. Cell 1991; 67: 1–20

22 Pergolizzi RG, Erster SH, Goonewardena P, Brown WT. Detection of the full fragile X mutation. Lancet 1992; 339: 271–272

23 Richards RI, Holman K, Kozman H et al. Fragile X syndrome: genetic localization by linkage mapping of two microsatellite repeats FRAXAC1 and FRAXAC2 which immediately flank the fragile site. J Med Genet 1991; 28: 818–823

24 Hirst M, Knight S, Cross G et al. Prenatal diagnosis of the fragile X syndrome. Lancet 1991; 338: 956–957

25 Sutherland GR, Gedeon A, Kornman L et al. Prenatal diagnosis of the fragile X syndrome. N Engl J Med 1991; 325: 1720–1722

26 Rousseau F, Heitz D, Biancalana V et al. Direct detection by DNA analysis of the fragile X syndrome of mental retardation. N Engl J Med 1991; 325: 1673–1681

27 Worhle D, Rott H-D, Kotzot D et al. Microdeletion of less than 250kb including the proximal part of the FMR-1 gene and the fragile site, in a male with the clinical phenotype of fragile X syndrome. Am J Hum Genet 1992; 52: 290–306

28 Gedeon AK, Baker E, Robinson H et al. Fragile X syndrome without CCG amplification has an FMR-1 deletion. Nature Genet 1992; 1: 341–344

29 De Boulle K, Verkerk JMH, Reyniers E et al. A point mutation in the FMR-1 gene associated with fragile X mental retardation. Nature Genet 1993; 3: 31–35

30 Sutherland G, Baker E. Characterisation of a new rare fragile site easily confused with the fragile X. Hum Mol Genet 1992; 1: 111–113

31 Flynn G, Hirst M, Knight S et al. The identification of the FRAXE site in two families ascertained for X linked mental retardation. J Med Genet 1993; 30: 97–100

32 Hirst MC, Barnicoat A, Flynn G et al. The identification of a third fragile site, FRAXF, in Xq27-q28 distal to both FRAXA and FRAXE. Hum Mol Genet 1993; 2: 197–200

33 La Spada AR, Fischbeck KH. Variant androgen receptor gene in X-linked spinal and bulbar muscular atrophy. Nature 1991; 352: 77–79

34 Brook J, McCurrach M, Harley H et al. Molecular basis of myotonic dystrophy: expansion of a trinucleotide (CTG) repeat at the 3′ end of a transcript encoding a protein kinase family member. Cell 1992; 68: 799–808

35 Worhle A, Hirst M, Davies K, Steinbach P. Genotype variation in fragile X fetal tissues. Hum Genet 1992; 89: 114–116

36 Brown WT. The fragile X: progress toward solving the puzzle. Am J Hum Genet 1990; 47: 175–180

37 Vogel F, Crusio WE, Kovac C et al. Selective advantage of fra(X) heterozygotes. Hum Genet 1990; 86: 25–32

38 Richards RI, Holman K, Friend K et al. Evidence of founder chromosomes in fragile X syndrome. Nature Genet 1992; 1: 257–260
39 Morton NE, MacPherson J. Population genetics of the fragile X syndrome: multi-allelic model for the FMR1 locus. Proc Natl Acad Sci (USA) 1992; 89: 4215–4217
40 Model B, Kuliev AM. A scientific basis for cost-benefit analysis of genetics services. Trends Genet 1993; 9: 46–52

10

Recent advances in sickle cell disease

G. R. Serjeant

BACKGROUND

Sickle cell disease is a generic term implying a disease process attributable to the presence of sickle haemoglobin (HbS) The term embraces several distinct genotypes, of which homozygous sickle cell (SS) disease and sickle cell-haemoglobin C (SC) disease are generally the most common. Less common genotypes include sickle cell-beta$^+$ (Sβ^+) thalassaemia and sickle cell-beta$^\circ$ (Sβ°) thalassaemia. Rare genotypes giving rise to sickle cell disease include sickle cell-haemoglobin D Punjab disease, sickle cell-haemoglobin O Arab disease and sickle cell-haemoglobin Lepore Washington. The relative frequency of these conditions is determined by the gene frequency in the population, the age structure of the population and their relative mortality. At the main government hospital in Kingston, Jamaica, SS disease occurs once in every 300 births, SC disease once in 500 births, Sβ^+ thalassaemia once in 3000 births and Sβ° thalassaemia once in 7000 births.[1] Other genotypes are much less frequent. The same pathological processes are common to all genotypes but vary in frequency and severity. Of the major genotypes, the most severe are SS disease and Sβ° thalassaemia, whereas SC disease and Sβ^+ thalassaemia are mild, although there is great clinical variability even within SS disease. The following chapter deals essentially with SS disease, although most of the lessons apply to a lesser extent to other genotypes. Where other genotypes have particular features, these will be stressed.

NATURAL HISTORY

Past observations of sickle cell disease have been biased towards severely affected cases and there is a false impression of the severity of the disease. Hospital experience focuses on a small group of severely affected individuals requiring frequent hospital admission, whereas mildly affected cases may not even attend hospital clinics. This reservation must be borne in mind when discussing prognosis or genetic counselling in this condition. In addition, there can be little doubt that the outcome and expression of the disease have also changed as a result of more effective therapy and management over the past 20 years. Current concepts of SS disease are therefore changing and this should influence the approach to the disease by both the patient and society at large. Since much of the morbidity and mortality of sickle cell disease occurs in the first 3 years of life and especially the first year, early diagnosis is essential in order to implement prophylactic programmes.

DIAGNOSIS

Antenatal diagnosis

The diagnosis of SS disease may now be made in the first 8–10 weeks of pregnancy,[2] offering the option of termination of pregnancy. Fetal material may be obtained either by chorionic villus sampling (CVS) or by amniocentesis. CVS may be performed as early as 6–8 weeks of pregnancy, although recent concerns that early CVS may cause fetal malformations have favoured delay in this procedure until 10 weeks. It may be performed by either the vaginal or transabdominal route, the latter having a lower risk of infection. Amniocentesis may also be performed as early as 10 weeks but the small amount of DNA obtained requires amplification by the polymerase chain reaction. The technical expertise for amniocentesis is more widely available than that for CVS, which also carries a greater risk of fetal death (approximately 2% in most experienced laboratories) than amniocentesis. Both procedures require relatively sophisticated DNA technology, are expensive and are hardly applicable on a population-wide basis.

Neonatal diagnosis

This procedure is cheap, accurate and eminently suitable for population screening and offers the option for early introduction of prophylactic programmes. A variety of technical procedures are available but electrophoresis on cellulose acetate followed by confirmation on agar gel is most widely used. Blood samples may be obtained from the umbilical cord or by heelprick and dried samples on filter paper may be sent by post to a central laboratory. The diagnosis should always be confirmed by repeating the procedure after 2–3 months.

SPLENIC DYSFUNCTION SYNDROMES

Pneumococcal septicaemia

Consequent on the early impairment of splenic function, there is an increased susceptibility to pneumococcal septicaemia, especially in the first 3 years of life.[3] The earliest reported cases have been at 4 months of age, so prophylaxis should commence as early as possible. Penicillin prevents infection, whether given intramuscularly in depot preparations[3] or orally,[4] but also prevents naturally acquired immunity so that stopping penicillin without vaccine cover may be followed by an increased incidence of septicaemia.[3] The main problem with oral penicillin is ensuring compliance. The pneumococcal vaccine induces poor antibody levels to some pneumococcal serotypes, especially before the age of 2 years and so confers incomplete protection before this age. The efficacy of penicillin has led to recommendations of lifelong prophylaxis and a study is currently underway in the USA comparing discontinuing penicillin at the age of 5 years with lifelong coverage. Penicillin should start as early as possible — preferably before 4 months — and continue for at least 4–5 years. It should not be stopped until at least 1 month after the 23 valent vaccine is given.

If targeting of a particularly susceptible population is necessary, there is some evidence that children who develop a palpable spleen within the first 6 months of life are at highest risk of developing subsequent pneumococcal septicaemia.[5]

Acute splenic sequestration

Sudden splenic enlargement with trapping of a large proportion of the red cell mass, resulting in the rapid onset of profound anaemia (Hb<4 g/dl) and a compensatory reticulocytosis, is an important cause of early morbidity and mortality. In the Jamaican cohort study, acute splenic sequestration was the major cause of mortality before 2 years of age. The aetiology of the episodes is unknown, although low fetal haemoglobin (HbF) levels are a risk factor[6] consistent with greater sickling. The haematological dynamics are consistent with a sudden obstruction of splenic outflow, and the resolution of splenomegaly either spontaneously or following transfusion implies that the splenic obstruction is reversible. In the absence of other known risk or precipitating factors, prevention is not possible and treatment of the acute episode entails immediate transfusion. Following transfusion, the introduction into the circulation of red cells from both the transfusion and the spleen as it diminishes in size may result in unexpectedly high haemoglobin levels.

Episodes of acute splenic sequestration tend to recur at increasingly frequent intervals[7] and prophylactic splenectomy is usually recommended after 2 attacks. The mortality of the initial attack of acute splenic sequestration has been markedly reduced by parental education in splenic palpation allowing earlier presentation to hospital for transfusion.[7]

Chronic hypersplenism

Sustained splenic enlargement with chronic red cell destruction and compensatory marrow expansion may result in a new haematological equilibrium with haemoglobin levels between 3 and 6 g/dl and reticulocytes generally exceeding 20%. This syndrome of hypersplenism is associated with a greatly expanded bone marrow, high demands for available protein and calories, and interference with growth which may accelerate following splenectomy. The high metabolic demands, the morbidity of coping with very low haemoglobin levels, the dangers of superimposed acute splenic sequestration or aplastic crisis, and the possibility of haemorrhage from thrombocytopenia argue for earlier intervention than the traditional treatment by chronic transfusion while awaiting possible spontaneous resolution. Some cases of hypersplenism do resolve spontaneously, but the greater morbidity of affected children in Jamaica has led to a policy of splenectomy if the condition persists for more than 6 months.

CONSEQUENCES OF HAEMOLYSIS

Aplastic crisis

The aplastic crisis is another cause of acute anaemia which may lead to readily preventable mortality in young children. Caused by human parvovirus (B19) infection,[8] there is a total destruction of red cell precursors manifested by absence of reticulocytes from the peripheral blood and a daily fall in haemoglobin level, the rate determined by the red cell survival. The aplasia is always self-limiting with a mean duration of 7–10 days but by the time of clinical presentation, the haemoglobin is often 2–4 g/dl and urgent transfusion is required. The clinical course is so predictable that in the absence of other complications, transfusion may be performed as an outpatient procedure with subsequent daily monitoring to ensure that the expected reticulocytosis occurs. Recurrent aplastic crises from B19 infection have never been described and immunity appears to be lifelong. A vaccine against B19 is currently under development and, if successful, may remove the aplastic crisis as a complication of SS disease.

Megaloblastic change

The accelerated erythropoiesis in SS disease increases demands for folic acid and the risks of consequent megaloblastic change depend on the dietary availability of this vitamin. In West Africa, megaloblastic change from folate deficiency in SS disease is common, whereas in Jamaica dietary folate is high and megaloblastic change is uncommon, although disappearance of folate-rich foods during natural disasters may be followed by a sudden increase in deficiency.[9] A controlled trial of folate supplementation in the Jamaican Cohort Study during the period of especially high demand (age 2–6 years) failed to show differences in haematology or growth between folate- and placebo-treated groups,[10] consistent with the relative infrequency of folate deficiency in unsupplemented patients in Jamaica. The place of folate supplementation should be determined by local conditions but is logical at times of rapid growth in infancy, adolescence and pregnancy. Patients should not be made psychologically dependent on folic acid.

Megaloblastic change is manifest haematologically by a slow progressive fall in haemoglobin level which may not cause symptoms until levels of 2–3 g/dl are reached, associated with reticulocyte counts below steady-state levels and an increasing mean cell volume (MCV). The latter typically exceeds 100 fl but may be difficult to interpret in the absence of steady-state data for the individual patient. Genetically determined microcytosis (e.g. SS disease with alpha-thalassaemia or Sβ° thalassaemia) may mask megaloblastic change, the MCV only increasingly from 65 to 85 fl, whereas other patients with high HbF levels may manifest MCV levels of 105–110 fl as steady-state values without megaloblastic change. Megaloblastic change is treated by oral folate which induces a rapid reticulocytosis and a gradual and progressive increase in haemoglobin level. Transfusion is rarely necessary, even at very low haemoglobin levels.

Gallstones

Rapid haemolysis and increased bilirubin excretion result in an increased prevalence of gallstones in SS disease which have been reported as early as 2 years of age. In the Jamaican cohort study, the incidence reached 33% by the age of 15–17 years and, of 62 children with gallstones, only 1 has developed specific symptoms — an empyema requiring cholecystectomy. Non-specific abdominal pain is significantly more frequent in the children with gallstones, but both gallstones and abdominal pain independently reflect severity of the disease and do not appear to be causally related.[11] Cholecystectomy is indicated for specific symptoms such as acute cholecystitis or obstruction of the common bile duct, but the role of prophylactic removal of asymptomatic gallstones is controversial.

BONE PROBLEMS

Dactylitis and painful crises

The metabolically active bone marrow is prone to ischaemia if the blood supply is reduced by either vaso-occlusion or shunting. Death of bone marrow initiates an inflammatory response, increasing intramedullary pressure, pain and swelling over the affected bones. In young children the process is most marked in the small bones of the hands and feet and is manifest as the hand-foot syndrome or dactylitis.

Dactylitis is often the first manifestation, occurring as early as 3–4 months, and is pathognomonic of SS disease, leading to the initial diagnosis when not already established by neonatal screening. The prevalence reaches 50% by the age of 2 years and then declines, being rare after the age of 5 years. Attacks frequently recur but resolution is usually clinically and radiologically complete, although damage to the growing epiphysis, possibly from infection, may cause premature fusion and permanent shortening of the affected small bones. Treatment is by pain relief and reassurance of the mother.

Dactylitis is the paediatric counterpart of the painful crisis and disappears coincident with the removal of active bone marrow from the small bones of the hands and feet. In older children and adults the pain distribution reflects the new distribution of active marrow in the flat bones and juxta-articular areas of the long bones. Pain most commonly affects bones adjacent to the knee, the pelvis and the lumbosacral spine. Precipitating factors include cold exposure, infection, severe exercise, emotional stress, and pregnancy, of which the most common in Jamaica is cold exposure. The frequency of painful crises increases during adolescence in males but not females.[12] Haematological risk factors include a high total haemoglobin[12,13] and low HbF.[13] Painful crises are more common in genotypes with less intravascular sickling such as SS disease with homozygous alpha-thalassaemia and Sβ° thalassaemia, casting doubt on the aetiological role of sickling-induced vaso-occlusion. This observation, the frequency of symmetrical, bilateral involvement, and the precipitation by skin cooling have given rise to the hypothesis that painful crises may result from a centrally mediated reflex shunting of blood away from the bone marrow.[14]

Management is based on avoidance of known precipitating factors, treatment of underlying infection if present, rehydration where necessary, warmth, reassurance and pain relief. There is some evidence that patient-controlled analgesia results in better pain control with lower overall doses of narcotic analgesia.[15]

Avascular necrosis of bone and osteomyelitis

The painful crisis is due to avascular necrosis of limited areas of active bone marrow, but occasionally larger areas may be affected, resulting in the clinical syndrome of avascular necrosis of bone with swelling and marked tenderness of the affected area. The upper third of the tibia is a common site and occasionally an entire bone, such as the humerus may be affected. Treatment consists of pain relief as in the painful crisis, although systemic symptoms may be more marked, raising concerns of underlying osteomyelitis. Differentiation of avascular necrosis of bone from osteomyelitis may be difficult, even with sophisticated radionuclide scans,[16] and in the absence of confirmatory evidence such as positive blood cultures, empirical treatment with antibiotics is justified. Since the commonest organisms causing osteomyelitis are *Salmonella* species, the most appropriate antibiotics are ampicillin, co-trimoxazole or chloramphenicol.

Femoral head necrosis

Avascular necrosis of bone marrow within the femoral head leads to special complications because of weight-bearing at this site. The clinical pattern depends on the age at which femoral head necrosis occurs. Involvement of the immature capital epiphysis results in flattening and remodelling of the femoral head which retains good function and rarely requires surgery. Involvement of the mature capital epiphysis produces segmental collapse with marked pain and limitation of movement and, although symptoms may resolve completely, surgical remodelling or total hip replacement may be required. Early diagnosis is essential to prevent severe deformity and magnetic resonance imaging may detect changes well before conventional radiography.[17] Initial treatment is based on avoidance of weight-bearing by crutches (or traction if the latter is impossible) for 4–6 months but persistent symptoms may require reconstructive surgery. Total hip replacement should be considered only if the patient is incapacitated by symptoms.

ABDOMINAL PAINFUL CRISIS

The abdominal painful crisis occurs predominantly in childhood. Pain may be referred from the spine or ribs but there is a particularly characteristic syndrome with diffuse tenderness, abdominal distention, reduced or absent bowel sounds, ileus, and sometimes fluid levels on radiology. The mechanism is unknown but is consistent with a localized area of bowel dysfunction. The syndrome usually resolves spontaneously after 3–5 days on conservative management and surgical exploration should be avoided unless there are clear surgical indications.

ACUTE CHEST SYNDROME

Attacks of pleuritic pain, shortness of breath, and clinical or radiological evidence of pulmonary pathology are common in SS disease and are usually referred to as the acute chest syndrome because the pathology is unclear. It is a common and serious problem, representing the largest single cause of mortality in SS disease at all ages after 2 years[18] and a major risk factor for chronic lung disease.[19] Most events probably have a combination of infection, infarction and pulmonary sequestration. Episodes in childhood were believed to be predominantly infective but recent studies have isolated organisms in only 4–14% of children.[20] The poor response to antibiotics and the dramatic resolution in some cases following transfusion[21] support a vascular rather than infective aetiology. Treatment usually consists of broad-spectrum antibiotics which, even in the absence of a primary infection, may have the advantage of preventing secondary infection. Severe episodes should be monitored by pulse oximetry and blood gas analysis. Deterioration in pulmonary function with falling oxygen saturation should be treated as an emergency and may be dramatically reversed by exchange transfusion.[22]

GROWTH

Height and weight are reduced in children with SS disease and puberty is delayed.[23] A deficit in mean weight occurs as early as 2 years of age and persists throughout life. The reduced mean height occurs from 1 year of age, increases during childhood and is further accentuated during puberty, which is reached later in SS disease than in normal children. Epiphyseal fusion terminates longitudinal bone growth in normal adolescents, but delayed fusion allows growth to continue for longer in SS patients and the height difference narrows, the mean final height in SS disease exceeding normal. The cause of these growth abnormalities is unknown, although observations in hypersplenism in which growth slows or stops and accelerates following splenectomy raise the possibility that erythropoietic expansion may, in some way, be causally related. The metabolic rate is increased in SS disease[24,25] and increases further in hypersplenism, consistent with the concept that growth abnormalities reflect the metabolic cost of bone marrow expansion. The delay in sexual development − on average 2.5 years in onset of menarche − is commensurate with the delay in physical development. Parents and patients should be informed and reassured about this different growth pattern and pubertal delay so that they may avoid wasting resources on 'tonics' to help the child gain weight.

LEG ULCERATION

Ulceration of the skin around the ankles affects up to 75% of Jamaican SS patients[26] but only 5% of those in the USA.[27] In Jamaica, ulcers develop most frequently between the ages of 15 and 20 years, approximately half follow trauma and half are spontaneous with characteristics suggestive of skin infarction. Typically ulcers heal slowly and readily break down, the healing/relapsing course continuing for as long as 10–20 years. Active therapy of early ulcers may expedite healing and reduce the chances of recurrence so small ulcers around the ankles should be taken seriously. Treatment is unsatisfactory and based on regular cleaning and debridement, bed rest, oral zinc sulphate, and firm supportive elastic bandages. Skin grafting is disappointing and subject to a high recurrence rate.

NOCTURNAL ENURESIS

Enuresis is a distressing complication rarely studied because of its benign nature and tendency to spontaneous resolution. Defined as wet at least 2 nights per week at the age of 8 years, enuresis occurred in 45% of children with SS disease, 15% with SC disease, and in 19% of controls with a normal haemoglobin (AA) genotype followed in the same cohort study.[28] Enuretic subjects tended to have higher urinary volumes and lower maximum functional bladder capacities and the ratio of urinary volume to maximum functional bladder capacity was significantly higher than in non-enuretic age/sex/genotype-matched controls.[29] These observations suggest that enuretic alarms may be the most appropriate method of intervention with the intention of converting nocturnal enuresis into nocturia.

STROKE

Major cerebrovascular episodes and stroke are devastating complications in SS disease, occurring predominantly in childhood with frequent recurrence within 3 years of the initial episode.[30] The incidence in the Jamaican cohort study was 8% by 14 years, with most occurring between 3 and 10 years.[31] Approximately 80% are associated with partial or complete blocks of major cerebral vessels[32] and recognized risk factors include acute anaemia, painful crises, a preceding high white cell count[31] and possibly low HbF levels.[30] The possible predictive roles of cerebral vessel stenosis detected by transcranial Doppler[33] and of sleep apnoea[34] are being explored. Treatment is currently unsatisfactory and based on prevention of recurrences by chronic transfusion programmes. The necessary duration is unknown but recurrences have followed cessation after 10–12 years. Other problems associated with chronic transfusion are iron overload, which requires chelation therapy, delayed transfusion reactions and blood-born infections.

PROLIFERATIVE SICKLE RETINOPATHY

Vaso-occlusion in the peripheral retina causes ischaemia and retinal infarction which induces attempts at revascularization. The resulting proliferative sickle retinopathy (PSR) may impair vision transiently by vitreous haemorrhage or permanently by retinal detachment. Peripheral retinal vessel occlusion may be observed from 5 years of age and PSR from 7 years.[35] PSR predominates in the more mild SC genotype, which accounted for 17 of 18 affected adolescents in the Jamaican cohort study. Treatment of PSR lesions by laser photocoagulation significantly reduces the risk of visual loss[36] but spontaneous autoinfarction is also common. Although PSR may eventually affect 75% of adults with SC disease, visual loss is rare and more knowledge is needed on the determinants of outcome of PSR before the role of laser treatment can be defined.

MORTALITY

Morbidity and mortality are low in the first 6 months, probably because of high HbF levels, but the highest risk period is between 6 months and 1 year of life: mortality tends to fall for each successive year afterwards. The causes of death are age-specific and early deaths result from acute splenic sequestration, pneumococcal septicaemia, and the acute chest syndrome (Table 10.1). In the Jamaican cohort study, mortality in SS disease was 5.8% in the

Table 10.1   Causes of 65 deaths in the Jamaican cohort study. (Reproduced with permission from Serjeant & Serjeant 1993.[41])

Age group (years)	No. of deaths	Causes
0–	17	ACS (6), ASS (5), Gastro (3), Pn sepsis (2), unknown (1)
1–	8	ACS (3), ASS (2), Pn sepsis (2) Gastro (1)
2–	7	ACS (2), ASS (2), Gastro (1), meningitis (1), unknown (1)
3–	2	Pn sepsis (1), unknown (1)
4–	3	ASS (1), CVA (1), unknown (1)
5–	4	Pn sepsis (3), *Salmonella* sepsis (1)
6–	3	Pn sepsis (1), H flu sepsis (1), aplasia (1)
7–	6	CVA (2), Pn sepsis (1), meningitis (1), MVA (1), unknown (1)
8–	1	*Salmonella* sepsis (1)
9–	2	CVA (1), MVA (1)
10–	1	Aplasia (1)
11–	0	
12–	2	ACS (2)
13–	3	ACS (1), CVA (1), portal vein thrombosis (1)
14–	2	CVA (2)
15–	3	ASS (1), CVA (1), glue sniffing (1)
16–	0	
17–	0	
18–	1	Pregnancy (1)

ACS = Acute chest syndrome; ASS = acute splenic sequestration; Gastro = gastroenteritis; Pn sepsis = pneumococcal septicaemia; MVA = motor vehicle accident; CVA = cerebrovascular accident; H flu = *Haemophilus influenzae*.

first year of life, 12.3% in the first 5 years, 17.6% by the age of 10 years and 25.9% by the age of 19 years (Fig. 10.1). Average life expectancy varies markedly in different environments, with different standards of medical care, and with the current age of the patient. By the age of 10 years, the high-risk period of early childhood has been passed and there may be excellent chances of surviving to 30–40 years of age. Survival is also likely to be improving rapidly as the causes of the high mortality in childhood are being addressed. In Jamaica, many patients with SS disease survive to 40–50 years, several patients are currently over 70 years and the longest survivor died recently at 77 years. The outlook has therefore improved dramatically and the best chances of surviving in good health are early diagnosis allowing implementation of prophylaxis against pneumococcal septicaemia and acute splenic sequestration and regular monitoring at experienced sickle cell clinics.

THE ROLE OF SICKLE CELL CLINICS

Patients with sickle cell disease require special services and expertise which are best administered through specialist clinics. Doctors and nurses specializing in the care of SS disease will be more adept at monitoring such patients, instructing families in the diagnosis of acute splenic sequestration, and reinforcing the need for penicillin prophylaxis. Regular review of patients even when clinically well documents the clinical and haematological

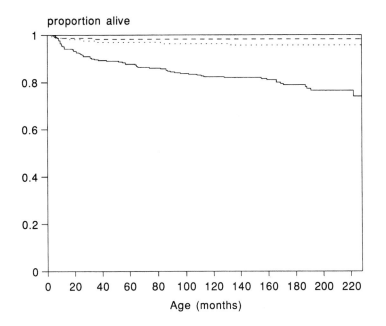

proportion alive

Fig. 10.1 Survival analysis from birth to 19 years (228 months) in the Jamaican cohort study. Continuous line = sickle cell disease; dotted line = sickle cell-haemoglobin C disease; dashed line = controls with a normal haemoglobin (AA) genotype followed in the same cohort study.

characteristics of the steady state against which changes during acute illnesses may be evaluated. Experienced observers, when faced with a severe anaemia, will know that the likely differential diagnosis is acute splenic sequestration, the aplastic crisis or megaloblastic change and will investigate and treat appropriately. Doctors familiar with the disease are unlikely to refer asymptomatic gallstones or the abdominal painful crisis for what may be unnecessary surgery. Specialized referral services, such as an ophthalmologist for laser treatment or vitreous surgery or an orthopaedic surgeon for total hip replacement, may be better provided by specialists linked to a sickle cell clinic and with an interest and experience in sickle cell disease, reducing judgement and management errors and avoiding unnecessary or inappropriate procedures.

NEWER APPROACHES TO THERAPY

There have been two major recent developments in relation to therapy of the disease; drug-induced increase in HbF levels and bone marrow transplantation.

High levels of HbF ameliorate many of the manifestations of sickle cell disease and this has been achieved by 5-azacytidine,[37] hydroxyurea[38] and sodium butyrate.[39] There are concerns on the optimal level of HbF to be achieved and on the fact that patient populations with mean HbF levels as high as 15–20% in the Eastern Province of Saudi Arabia and Central India still have significant complications from their disease. This work is still experimental and some of the agents are potentially toxic although hydroxyurea is currently under clinical trial in the USA. These agents should not be used as routine clinical therapy until more information is available on their efficacy and potential side-effects.

Bone marrow transplantation has the potential to cure the disease but its clinical place depends on the relative risks of the procedure and of the underlying disease. The risks of the procedure have diminished, but the inability to predict a severe clinical course in SS disease limits its application. Its use in SS disease[40] remains controversial and the high cost and technical expertise required imply that it is unlikely to be widely available within the foreseeable future.

KEY POINTS FOR CLINICAL PRACTICE

- Neonatal diagnosis is essential for prophylaxis of early complications.
- Prophylactic penicillin prevents pneumococcal septicaemia.
- Parental education reduces mortality from acute splenic sequestration.
- Reticulocyte counts are essential for interpretation of acute anaemic episodes.
- Gallstones rarely cause symptoms.
- Folate supplementation is cheap and harmless but do not make your patients psychologically dependent.
- Treat minor abrasions around the ankles seriously, as they may become chronic leg ulcers.
- Magnetic resonance imaging may be helpful in the early diagnosis of femoral head necrosis.
- Clinical services for sickle cell disease management are best coordinated through specialized sickle cell clinics.

REFERENCES

1 Serjeant GR, Serjeant BE, Forbes M, Hayes RJ, Higgs DR, Lehmann H. Haemoglobin gene frequencies in the Jamaican population: a study in 100 000 newborns. Br J Haematol 1986; 64: 253–262
2 Old JM, Fitches A, Heath C et al. First-trimester fetal diagnosis for haemoglobinopathies: report 200 cases. Lancet 1986: ii: 763–768
3 John AB, Ramlal A, Jackson H, Maude GH, Waight-Sharma A, Serjeant GR. Prevention of pneumococcal infection in children with homozygous sickle cell disease. Br Med J 1984; 288: 1567–1570
4 Gaston MH, Verter JI, Woods G et al. Prophylaxis with oral penicillin in children with sickle cell anemia. N Engl J Med 1986; 314: 1593–1599
5 Rogers DW, Vaidya S, Serjeant GR. Early splenomegaly in homozygous sickle-cell disease: an indicator of susceptibility to infection. Lancet 1978; ii: 963–965
6 Stevens MCG, Hayes RJ, Vaidya S, Serjeant GR. Fetal hemoglobin and clinical severity of

homozygous sickle cell disease in early childhood. J Pediatr 1981; 98: 37–41

7 Emond AM, Collis R, Darvill D, Higgs DR, Maude GH, Serjeant GR. Acute splenic sequestration in homozygous sickle cell disease: natural history and management. J Pediatr 1985; 107: 201–206

8 Serjeant GR, Topley JM, Mason K et al. Outbreak of aplastic crises in sickle cell anaemia associated with parvovirus-like agent. Lancet 1981; 2: 595–597

9 Readett DRJ, Serjeant BE, Serjeant GR. Hurricane Gilbert anaemia. Lancet 1989; 2: 101–102

10 Rabb LM, Grandison Y, Mason K, Hayes RJ, Serjeant BE, Serjeant GR. A trial of folate supplementation in children with homozygous sickle cell disease. Br J Haematol 1983; 54: 589–594

11 Webb DKH, Darby JS, Dunn DT, Terry SI, Serjeant GR. Gallstones in Jamaican children with homozygous sickle cell disease. Arch Dis Child 1989; 64: 693–696

12 Baum KF, Dunn DT, Maude GH, Serjeant GR. The painful crisis of homozygous sickle cell disease: a study of risk factors. Arch Intern Med 1987; 147: 1231–1234

13 Platt OS, Thorington BD, Brambilla DJ et al. Pain in sickle cell disease. Rates and risk factors. N Engl J Med 1991; 325: 11–16

14 Serjeant GR, Chalmers RM. Is the painful crisis of sickle cell disease a 'steal' syndrome? J Clin Pathol 1990; 43: 789–791

15 McPherson E. Perlin E, Finke H, Castro O, Pittman J. Patient-controlled analgesia in patients with sickle cell vaso-occlusive crisis. Am J Med Sci 1990; 229: 10–12

16˙ Kim HC, Alavi A, Russell MO, Schwartz E. Differentiation of bone and bone marrow infarcts from osteomyelitis in sickle cell disorders. Clin Nucl Med 1989; 14: 249–254

17 Rao VM. Mitchell DG, Steiner RM et al. Femoral head avascular necrosis in sickle cell anemia: MR characteristics: Magn Reson Imaging 1988; 6: 661–667

18 Thomas AN, Pattison C, Serjeant GR. Causes of death in sickle cell disease in Jamaica. Br Med J 1982: 285: 633–635

19 Powars DR, Weidman JA, Odom-Maryon T, Niland JC, Johnson C. Sickle cell chronic lung disease: prior morbidity and the risk of pulmonary failure. Medicine 1988; 67: 66–76

20 Sprinkle RH, Cole T, Smith S, Buchanan GR. Acute chest syndrome in children with sickle cell disease. A retrospective analysis of 100 hospitalized cases. Am J Pediatr Hematol/Oncol 1986; 8: 105–110

21 Davies SC, Luce PJ, Win AA, Riordan JF, Brozovic M. Acute chest syndrome in sickle cell disease. Lancet 1984; i: 36–38

22 Lanzkowsky P, Shende A, Karayalcin G, Kim YJ, Aballi AJ. Partial exchange transfusion in sickle cell anemia. Am J Dis Child 1978; 132: 1206–1208

23 Stevens MCG, Maude GH, Cupidore L, Jackson H, Hayes RJ, Serjeant GR. Prepubertal growth and skeletal maturation in sickle cell disease. Pediatrics 1986; 78: 124–132

24 Badaloo A, Jackson AA, Jahoor F. Whole body protein turnover and resting metabolic rate in homozygous sickle cell disease. Clin Sci 1989; 77: 93–97

25 Singhal A, Davies P, Sahota A, Thomas PW, Serjeant GR. Resting metabolic rate in homozygous sickle cell disease. Am J Clin Nutr 1993; 57: 32–34

26 Serjeant GR. Leg ulceration in sickle cell anemia. Arch Intern Med 1974; 133: 690–694

27 Koshy M, Entsuah A, Koranda A et al. Leg ulcers in patients with sickle cell disease. Blood 1989; 74: 1403–1408

28 Readett DRJ, Morris JS, Serjeant GR. Nocturnal enuresis in sickle cell haemoglobinopathies. Arch Dis Child 1990; 65: 290–293

29 Readett DRJ, Morris JS, Serjeant GR. Determinants of nocturnal enuresis in homozygous sickle cell disease. Arch Dis Child 1990; 65: 615–618

30 Powars D, Wilson B, Imbus C, Pegelow C, Allen J. The natural history of stroke in sickle cell disease. Am J Med 1978; 65: 461–471

31 Balkaran B, Char G, Morris JS, Serjeant BE, Serjeant GR. Stroke in a cohort study of patients with homozygous sickle cell disease. J Pediatr 1992; 120: 360–366

32 Gerald B, Sebes JI, Langston JW. Cerebral infarction secondary to sickle cell disease: arteriographic findings. AJR 1980; 134: 1209–1212

33 Adams RJ, McKie V, Nichols F et al. The use of transcranial ultrasonography to predict stroke in sickle cell disease. N Engl J Med 1992; 326: 605–610

34 Robertson PL, Aldrich MS, Hanash SM, Goldstein GW. Stroke associated with obstructive sleep apnea in a child with sickle cell anemia. Ann Neurol 1988; 23: 614–616

35 Talbot JF, Bird AC, Maude GH, Acheson RW, Moriarty BJ, Serjeant GR. Sickle cell retinopathy in Jamaican children: further observations from a cohort study. Br J Ophthalmol 1988; 72: 727–732
36 Farber MD, Jampol LM, Fox P et al, A randomized clinical trial of scatter photocoagulation of proliferative sickle cell retinopathy. Arch Ophthalmol 1991; 109: 363–367
37 Dover GJ, Charache S, Boyer SH, Vogelsang G, Moyer M. 5-Azacytidine increases HbF production and reduces anemia in sickle cell disease: dose–response analysis of subcutaneous and oral dosage regimens. Blood 1985; 66: 527–532
38 Rodgers GP, Dover GJ, Noguchi CT, Schechter AN, Nienhuis AW. Hematologic responses of patients with sickle cell disease to treatment with hydroxurea. N Engl J Med 1990; 322: 1037–1045
39 Perrine SP, Miller BA, Faller DV et al. Sodium butyrate enhances fetal globin gene expression in erythroid progenitors of patients with Hb SS and β thalassemia. Blood 1989; 74: 454–459
40 Ferster A, De Valek C, Azzi N, Fondu P, Toppet M, Sariban E. Bone marrow transplantation for severe sickle cell anaemia- Br J Haematol 1992; 80: 102–105
41 Serjeant GR, Serjeant BE. Management of sickle cell disease — lessons from the Jamaican Cohort Study. Blood Rev 1993; 7(3): 137–145

11

Fatty acids in human and formula milk

S. M. Innis

This review will describe recent advances in the understanding of infant lipid nutrition with regard to the composition, digestion, absorption and metabolism of human milk and formula fats, the role of specific fatty acids in growth and development, and the special needs of premature infants.

FATTY ACID NOMENCLATURE AND METABOLISM

Nomenclature

Fatty acids are usually referred to using a shorthand notation which gives the number of carbon atoms followed by a colon, then the number of unsaturated bonds and a notation n (or ω) with a number to designate the fatty acid series (Fig. 11.1, Table 11.1). The position of the first double bond from the methyl (*n*) terminus is used to designate the series of unsaturated fatty acids. Fatty acid metabolism may involve chain elongation (addition of 2 carbon units) or desaturation (insertion of double bonds between adjacent carbon atoms;

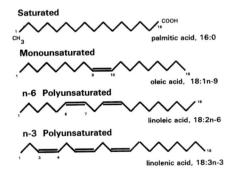

Fig. 11.1 Schematic representation of fatty acids to illustrate saturated, monounsaturated, n-6 and n-3 fatty acid families. CH_3, methyl, n (or ω) terminus; COOH, carboxyl (Δ) terminus. Fatty acid families are referred to by the position of the first double bond from methyl (n) terminus, i.e. n-9, n-6, n-3.

Table 11.1   Common names, abbreviations and melting points of fatty acids

Common or systematic name	Nomenclature	Melting point (°C)
Caproic	6:0	− 2
Caprylic	8:0	16.5
Capric	10:0	31.5
Lauric	12:0	44.0
Myristic	14:0	58.0
Palmitic	16:0	63.1
Stearic	18:0	71.2
Oleic	18:1	16.3
Linoleic	18:2n–6	− 5.0
Linolenic	18:3n–3	− 11.3
Arachidonic	20:4n–6	− 49.5
Eicosapentaenoic	20:5n–3	− 53.5
Docosahexaenoic	22:6n–3	− 44.3

Fig. 11.2). The notation Δ is used to indicate the position from the carboxyl terminal, and the name of the enzyme, where a double bond is inserted.

Saturated fatty acids are usefully classified according to chain length as medium chain fatty acids, caprylic acid (8:0), capric acid (10:0) and lauric acid (12:0), intermediate chain length, myristic acid (14:0) and long chain fatty acids, fatty acids with 16 or more carbon atoms. The major long chain saturated fatty acids synthesized by mammalian tissues are palmitic acid (16:0) and stearic acid (18:0).

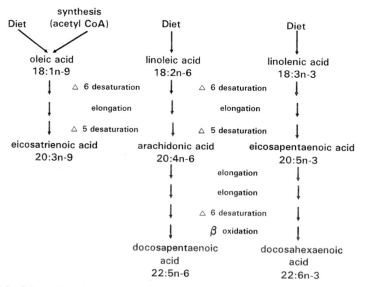

Fig. 11.2   Schematic representation of the major pathways of desaturation and elongation of oleic acid (18:1n–9), linoleic acid (18:2n–6) and linolenic acid (18:3n–3). Substrate preference of the $\Delta 6$ desaturase is in order 18:3n-3> 18:2n – 6>18:1, thus desaturation of 18:1 to eicosatrienoic acid (20:3n–9) occurs at appreciable rates only during deficiency of 18:2n–6 and 18:3n–3.

The major dietary lipid is triglyceride; this is a three-carbon alcohol (glycerol) which has one fatty acid esterified to each of three hydroxyl groups (Fig. 11.3). When the hydroxyl group at carbon three is linked to phosphoric acid and a polar group, the lipid is termed a phospholipid (e.g phosphatidylcholine, phosphatidylethanolamine). A bilayer of phospholipids, in which the fatty acids are oriented inwards to create a hydrophobic core, forms the structural matrix of all cell membranes. The physical properties and specific effects of certain fatty acids influence a variety of membrane functions, such as membrane transport, enzyme and receptor activities.

Dietary essential n-6 and n-3 fatty acids

Mammalian cells do not have the enzymes necessary to synthesize n-6 or n-3 polyunsaturated fatty acids.[1] Since these fatty acids have essential metabolic roles, a source of n-6 and n-3 fatty acids must be provided in the diet. The fatty acids known to be essential dietary nutrients are linoleic acid (18:2n-6) and linolenic acid (18:3n-3). Linoleic and linolenic acid can be further desaturated and elongated to more highly unsaturated, longer chain fatty acids (Fig. 11.2), of which arachidonic acid (20:4n-6), eicosapentaenoic acid (20:5n-3) and docosahexaenoic acid (22:6n-3) are particularly important. Small amounts of 20:4n-6, 22:5n-3 and 22:6n-3 are present in the diet as components of animal tissue lipids, and in human milk. The major dietary sources of linoleic acid (18:2n-6) and linolenic acid (18:3n-3) are plant and seed oils. Fats of vegetable origin, including infant formula with vegetable oils as the source of fat, contain no arachidonic, eicosapentaenoic or docosahexaenoic acid.[1-3]

Essential fatty acid metabolism

High intakes of linoleic acid (18:2n-6) can inhibit desaturation of linolenic acid (18:3n-3) to docosahexaenoic acid (22:6n-3) and conversely, high intakes of linolenic acid can inhibit synthesis of arachidonic acid (20:4n-6) from linoleic acid (18:2n-6).[1] This is explained by competition between 18:2n-6 and 18:3n-3 for the Δ6 desaturase enzyme. The desaturase enzymes are also sensitive to product inhibition, for example, desaturation of linoleic acid to arachidonic acid is inhibited by eicosapentaenoic acid (20:5n-3) and docosahexaenoic acid (22:6n-3). These aspects of fatty acid metabolism explain why the balance as well as amount of the different n-6 and n-3 fatty acids in the diet is important.

Fatty acids are also readily oxidized for energy, and can be incorporated into tissue triglycerides and cholesteryl esters. The use of fatty acids for energy, direct acylation into various lipids, or desaturation depends on the fatty acid chain length and unsaturation. Linoleic acid (18:2n-6) and linolenic acid (18:3n-3) are both efficiently oxidized for energy in the mitochondria.[1] Linoleic, but not linolenic acid, is incorporated in large amounts into

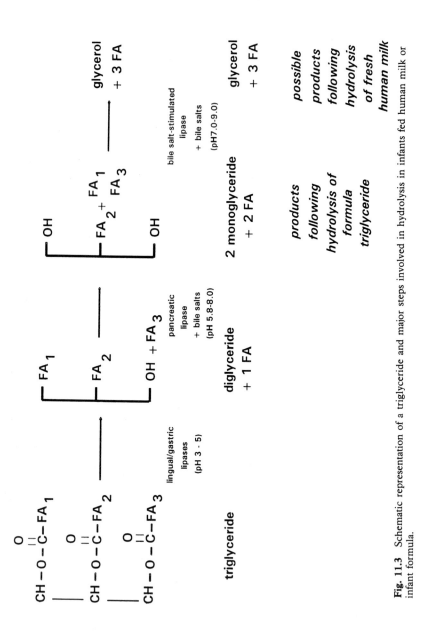

Fig. 11.3 Schematic representation of a triglyceride and major steps involved in hydrolysis in infants fed human milk or infant formula.

triglycerides and cholesteryl esters. Arachidonic (20:4n–6) and docosahexaenoic (22:6n–3) acid, on the other hand, are preferentially incorporated into membrane phospholipids and oxidation of 20:4n–6, 20:5n–3 and 22:6n–3 involves peroxisomal metabolism.[1] These differences in metabolism explain why dietary 18:2n–6 and 18:3n–3 are not equivalent to their respective metabolites, 20:4n–6 and 22:6n–3.

Essential fatty acid deficiency

Palmitic and stearic acid can be Δ9 desaturated to palmitoleic acid (16:1n–7) and oleic acid (18:1n–9), respectively. The Δ6 desaturase, however, has substrate preference for 18:3n–3 and 18:2n–6 over 18:1n–9. Because of this, desaturation of oleic acid (18:1) and elongation to eicosatrienoic acid (20:3n–9) proceed at appreciable rates only when the intake of linoleic and linolenic acid is below 1–2% energy (kcal).[1] An increase in the eicosatrienoic acid to arachidonic acid ratio, known as the triene : tetraene ratio, in plasma phospholipid or cholesteryl esters to 0.2 or higher is often used as the diagnostic criteria for essential fatty acid deficiency.[1]

N-6 AND N-3 FATTY ACIDS IN GROWTH AND DEVELOPMENT

Essential fatty acids and central nervous system (CNS) development

Research on fatty acid requirements during growth and development has been particularly concerned with the CNS. This is explained by the very high concentrations of arachidonic acid and docosahexaenoic acid in CNS membranes[4,5] and the knowledge that long-term functional problems may occur if fatty acid deficiency occurs during the period known as the brain growth spurt.[1] The human brain growth spurt commences at the beginning of the third trimester of gestation and continues for about 18 months after birth. Consistent with this, deposition of arachidonic (20:4n–6) and docosahexaenoic (22:6n–3) acid in the CNS is rapid and linear from about 28 weeks gestation and for several months after birth.[6]

Source of n-6 and n-3 fatty acids for the developing CNS

Considerable uncertainty surrounds the question of whether 20:4n–6 and 22:6n–3 are essential dietary nutrients for infants. CNS and other cells can synthesize arachidonic acid and docosahexaenoic acid from linoleic acid and linolenic acid, respectively, and the desaturase activity in the developing brain seems to be considerable.[1,7,8] The importance of CNS uptake of preformed arachidonic and docosahexaenoic acid from plasma, particularly during the third trimester of gestation, however, is not known.

Dietary requirements for n-6 and n-3 fatty acids for CNS development

Studies in other species have found altered learning behaviour and visual function, and reduced brain and retina docosahexaenoic acid (22:6n–3) as a result of feeding diets with less than 0.014% kcal linolenic acid (18:3n–3) during development.[1] The fatty acid-sufficient diets contained >0.3 per cent kcal 18:3n–3, usually from soybean oil, but no preformed docosahexaenoic acid. Maximum accretion of docosahexaenoic acid (22:6n–3) in rodent and piglet brain synaptic membranes and retina requires an intake of at least 0.7% kcal linolenic acid (18:3n–3).[1,9,10] Of note, the perinatal timing of the brain growth spurt and milk fatty acids are similar in piglets and infants. The intake of linoleic acid (18:2n–6) needed to support maximum levels of arachidonic acid (20:4n–6) in the developing CNS or other organs of rodents is relatively low – only about 3% kcal.[1,9] Intakes above 10–11% kcal (in a milk or formula, about 20% fatty acids), however, seem to reduce tissue 20:4n–6 and 22:6n–3. The optimum ratio of linoleic to linolenic acid (18:2n–6:18:3n–3) in the diet of young rodents or in formula-fed piglets seems to be 4:1 to 16:1, provided minimum requirements of both 18:2n–6 and 18:3n–3 are met. Similar data are not available for humans.

Although it seems that arachidonic and docosahexaenoic acid are not essential dietary nutrients for the term newborn in other species, including non-human primates,[1] similar direct information is not available for humans. Measurement of plasma or red blood cell phospholipid fatty acids has been widely used to assess fatty acid status in infants.[1,10,11] However, blood lipid n–6 and n–3 fatty acids reflect the amount of the fatty acid consumed in the diet, and not necessarily the amount synthesized, taken up or acylated into CNS tissues. Studies with infants, therefore, now combine analyses of blood fatty acids with measures of CNS functional development. Clinical studies are still hampered by the sparsity of information on the functional roles of 20:4n–6 and 22:6n–3 in CNS membranes. One exception is that retinal membrane concentrations of 22:6n–3 are known to be important to normal visual processes. Eighty per cent or more of the lipid in the retina rod outer segments is membrane phospholipid, and 22:6n–3 represents 40% or more of the total fatty acids.[4] Although the actual functional role of 22:6n–3 in the visual process is not yet clear, measures of visual development have become an integral part of many studies on the n–3 fatty acid requirements of infants.

COMPOSITION OF HUMAN MILK LIPIDS

Milk fat and cholesterol

Fat is the most variable macronutrient in human milk, varying with the stage of lactation, diurnally and within a feed.[3] Human milk usually contains about 3.5–4.5 g fat/dl, representing 40–55% milk kcal. The concentration is lower, often less than 2.0 g fat/dl, during the first week postpartum, then increases in the second week to the levels similar to mature milk.[12] Milk from women delivering prematurely has been found to have lower, similar or even higher fat contents than milk from women delivering at term.[12-14] Similarly, information on the effect of maternal high fat compared to high carbohydrate diets on milk fat is not consistent.[14,15]

Fat is secreted in milk as globules containing a core of triglycerides, representing about 98% milk total fat.[3] During secretion, the triglyceride becomes enveloped by the apical part of the phospholipid-rich membrane of the mammary gland epithelial cell. The membrane of phospholipids contains a higher percent arachidonic (20:4n–6) and docosahexaenoic (22:6n–3) acid than the milk triglycerides, but because phospholipids represent only 1.3% of the milk total fat, the quantitative contribution to total fatty acids is very low. Human milk contains about 20 mg cholesterol/dl with most present as the free sterol in the globule membrane. The amount of cholesterol in milk is not influenced by the maternal dietary cholesterol intake or hyperlipidaemia.[16,17]

Origin of milk fatty acids

The triglyceride fatty acids are derived from synthesis in the mammary alveolar cells and by uptake from plasma. The fatty acid composition of milk from women delivering prematurely and at term is generally similar. A total of about 185 different fatty acids have been identified.[3] These include a number of *trans* isomers and conjugated fatty acids, which probably originate from the mothers's diet. Concern over *trans* isomers of unsaturated fatty acids in human milk has been raised because the properties of *trans* isomers differ from those of naturally occurring *cis* isomers.[18] The major dietary sources of *trans* fatty acids are partially hydrogenated vegetable oils, and ruminant milk and tissue fats. Recent analysis of human milk in Germany found about 4% *trans* isomers.[18] Whether or not *trans* fatty acids are in any way detrimental to infant growth or development is not known.

Saturated fatty acids

Saturated fatty acids represent about 40% of the total fatty acids in milk.[23] Fatty acids synthesized by the mammary cells are shorter chain saturated fatty acids, lauric (12:0) and myristic (14:0) acid, and the proportion of these fatty acids in milk is increased by maternal high-carbohydrate diets.[19] This is probably explained by increased fatty acid synthesis from glucose in the mammary cells. The medium chain fatty acid, caprylic (8:0) and capric (10:0) acid are minor components, usually representing less than 2% milk fatty acids. Lauric and myristic acid represent about 10–12% fatty acids, and palmitic (16:0) and stearic (18:0) acid represent about 20% and 8% milk fatty acids, respectively in human milk. About 70% of the 16:0 is esterified to the centre (2) position of the milk triglyceride.[2,3] In other human and animal tissues (except lard) and vegetable oils, 16:0 is predominantly esterified to the outer (1,3) positions of the triglyceride.

n-6 and n-3 fatty acids

The n-6 and n-3 fatty acid content of human milk varies widely depending on the composition of fat in the mother's diet.[2,3] Levels of 18:2n–6 usually range from 8 to 16% fatty acids, but may be as high as 30% in milk from women following vegan diets.[20] An increase in 18:2n–6 in human milk during the last 2 decades, and higher levels in milk in the USA than Europe seems consistent with changes toward increasing use of polyunsaturated table fats and cooking oils. The ratio of linoleic acid (18:2n–6) to linolenic acid (18:3n–3) in human milk ranges from about 8:1 to over 45:1.[19] Human milk, however, contains preformed arachidonic (20:4n–6) and docosahexaenoic (22:6n–3) acid, thus the demands for endogenous synthesis of these fatty acids is not the same as in infants fed formulas containing 18:2n–6 and 18:3n–3 as the only n-6 and n-3 fatty acids.

The wide variation in docosahexaenoic acid (22:6n–3) in human milk is clearly explained by variations in maternal intake of animal and fish-derived fat.[2] Levels of 22:6n–3 from as low as 0.1% to as high as 1.4–1.5% have been found in the milk of women following vegan diets or diets high in marine fats, respectively.[2,19,20] Milk levels of arachidonic acid (20:4n–6) seem to be fairly constant at about 0.5% fatty acids. Whether this reflects the lack of extremes in maternal dietary intake, or regulation by the mammary gland is not known. The amounts of 20:4n–6 and 22:6n–3 in milk are not related to the milk content of 18:2n–6 or 18:3n–3. The differences in milk levels of n–6 and n–3 fatty acids are reflected in the blood lipids of breast-fed infants.[1,2,10,11,19,20] It is not known if variations in milk fatty acids due to maternal diet have any effect on growth and development of breast-fed infants.

DIGESTION AND ABSORPTION OF HUMAN MILK FAT

The coefficiency of fat absorption depends on gastrointestinal maturity, the composition of the fat, and any storage or processing of expressed human milk. The coefficiency of absorption of fat from fresh human milk is usually over 90%, even in small premature infants of less than 1500 g.[19,21] Malabsorption of fatty acids, if it occurs, may be significant, not only because of energy loss, but because it may result in malabsorption of important minerals such as calcium, and fat-soluble vitamins. The characteristics of human milk fat which confer the high coefficiency of absorption are thus of obvious relevance to the design of infant formula fat blends.

Fat hydrolysis by gastric and colipase-dependent pancreatic lipases

Fat digestion and absorption is the combined result of hydrolysis by several lipases and micelle formation in the aqueous phase of the intestine by bile salts (Fig. 11.3).[19,21,22] Initial hydrolysis of milk fat by gastric lipases is particularly important for continued triglyceride hydrolysis by colipase-dependent pancreatic lipase in the small intestine. The milk fat globule membrane of phospholipid, cholesterol and protein is relatively resistant to colipase-dependent pancreatic lipase.[19,22] Gastric lipases, however, can penetrate the globule membrane and initiate hydrolysis of the triglyceride core without disrupting the membrane. The free fatty acids formed induce binding between colipase-dependent pancreatic lipase and the globule, overcoming the resistance to hydrolysis. Gastric lipase have relatively low specific activity, are rapidly inactivated by pancreatic proteases in the presence of bile salts and are sensitive to product inhibition by free fatty acids. This suggests they do not play a major quantitative role in fat digestion.[22] Gastric lipase is present from about 26 weeks of gestation.[19,21] Whether low gastric lipase activity could limit hydrolysis of human milk fat in very premature infants is not known.

Milk bile salt-stimulated lipase

Human milk contains a lipase, bile salt-stimulated lipase, which is produced in the mammary gland and secreted in milk from about 26 weeks gestation.[21,22] Levels of the enzyme seem to be similar in preterm and term milk, and do not vary as a function of the length of lactation. Bile salt-stimulated lipase survives the acid enviroment of the stomach, has a pH optimum of 7–9 and, when mixed with bile salts, can hydrolyse a wide variety of triglycerides completely to glycerol and free fatty acids.[22] Pasteurization (63°C) of human milk leads to inactivation of bile salt-stimulated lipase, and reduces milk fat absorption to 75–90%.[19] The reduction in fat absorption could be explained by enzyme inactivation, favouring a quantitative role of bile salt-stimulated lipase in fat absorption. Other effects of heat processing, such as changes to the milk fat globule structure, are also possible.

Products of triglyceride digestion in infants fed milk and formula

Gastric and colipase-dependent pancreatic lipase are specific for fatty acids at the 1,3 positions of the triglyceride (Fig. 11.3).[19] Thus, the major products of triglyceride hydrolysis in infants fed formula are free fatty acids and 2-monoglycerides. Monoglycerides with palmitic acid (16:0) are micellarized and absorbed more readily than unesterified 16:0. The low absorption of unesterified 16:0 is related to a melting point above body temperature, which decreases solubility, and a tendency to form insoluble soaps with divalent cations, such as calcium, at the pH of the intestine. This explains why the absorption of 16:0 is higher from triglycerides with 16:0 at the 2, rather than the 1,3 position.[19,23] Continued hydrolysis of 2-monoglycerides from milk fat by the milk bile salt-stimulated lipase would release 16:0 from milk triglycerides. Such hydrolysis does not seem compatible with the high coefficiency of absorption of milk fat or the specific positioning of 16:0 at the

2 position of the milk triglycerides. The extent of 2-monoglyceride hydrolysis by bile salt-stimulated lipase in infants in vivo is not known.

COMPOSITION OF INFANT FORMULA LIPIDS

The composition of fatty acids in infant formulas varies widely depending on the type and proportions of vegetable and animal fats in the product. Selection of fat blends is usually based on physiological considerations of providing a well-absorbed and tolerated fat, adequate essential fatty acids, a composition resembling human milk, the absence of undesirable, potentially toxic compounds in the oil, and consumer acceptance.

Saturated fat sources

The coefficiency of absorption of unesterified fatty acids from the intestine decreases with increasing fatty acid chain length, but increases with increasing unsaturation. The coefffficiency of absorption of 8:0 and 10:0 is almost 100%, decreases to about 95% for 12:0, 89% for 14:0, 75% for 16:0 and 62% for 18:0, but increases again to over 90% for 18:1 and 18:2n-6.[24] This explains why saturated fatty acids with 8–14 carbons are often favoured over 16:0 and 18:0 in formula. The high coefficiency of absorption of medium chain fatty acids is explained by their solubility in water.[25] This decreases the dependence on bile salts for micellarization, and because hydrolysis of triglycerides with medium chain fatty acids is not obligatory for absorption, the requirement for lipase hydrolysis is also reduced. Medium chain triglycerides (MCT), which are semisynthetic oils prepared from coconut oil, with predominantly caprylic (8:0) and capric (10:0) acid, are, therefore, often used in formulas for premature or other infants in whom the bile salt pool or lipase activities may be low. Coconut oils, which contain predominantly lauric (12:0) and myristic (14:0) acid, are widely used in formulas for infants born after term gestation. Palm and beef oleo oils are high in 16:0, but over 80% is esterified to the 1,3 positions of the triglycerides.[3] As discussed, this is of potential concern with regard to fat and mineral absorption. The coefficiency of absorption of 16:0 is lower in infants fed formulas with these oils than in infants fed expressed human milk.[26] Lard and milk-derived fats contain a high proportion of 16:0, which is predominantly esterified to the 2 position of the triglyceride, more similar to human milk.

Unsaturated oil sources

Polyunsaturated oils such as corn, safflower and soybean oil are all well-absorbed, but are low in oleic acid (18:1n-9) and high in linoleic acid (18:2n-6). Corn, safflower and sunflower oils, and their high 18:1n-9 varieties are deficient in linolenic acid (18:3n-3), and have linoleic:linolenic acid ratios of 55:1 to over 250:1. If used, they should be blended with oils high in 18:3n–3, both to meet n–3 fatty acid requirements and to decrease the linoleic acid:linolenic acid ratio. Soybean, low erucic acid (22:1) rapeseed and Canola oils usually contain 6–8% 18:3n–3 and have linoleic acid:linolenic acid ratios of 3:1 to 9:1. Low erucic acid rapeseed, Canola and high oleic safflower and sunflower oil are rich in 18:1n–9, but low erucic acid and Canola oils are not approved for use in infant formulas in the USA. The low eruic acid rapeseed and Canola oils used for human consumption contain less than 2% erucic acid (22:1) and are not known to have any detrimental effects on health. The *trans* unsaturated fatty acid content of infant formula is usually less than in human milk; the highest amounts, 3–4.5% milk fatty acids, have been found in adapted formulas and home-made formulas based on fresh or evaporated cow-milk.[18]

Addition of arachidonic and/or docosahexaenoic acid

Formulas containing 20:4n–6 and/or 22:6n–3 have recently become available in· Europe and Asia. The 20:4n–6 and 22:6n–3 can be incorporated by including fish and/or egg total lipid or phospholipid in the fat blend. Docosahexaenoic acid (22:6n–3) is high in many fish oils, but is usually accompanied by high amounts of eicosapentaenoic acid (20:5n–3) and minimal 20:4n–6. Some tropical and very cold water fish contain high 22:6n–3 relative to 20:5n–3, and some have appreciable amounts of 20:4n–6. Depending on the fish oil, about 1–3% fat blend is needed to achieve an amount of 22:6n–3 similar to that in human milk. Egg total lipid is quite low in 20:4n–6 and 22:6n–3, requiring large amounts (15% or more) in the blend to attain levels of 20:4n–6 and 22:6n–3 comparable to milk; use of egg phospholipid requires amounts closer to 10% fat blend but the contribution of phosphorus is high. Depending on the extraction method, the egg lipid may or may not contribute significant amounts of cholesterol.

Cholesterol

Infants fed formulas with less than 5 mg cholesterol/dl have lower plasma total and low density lipoprotein cholesterol than infants fed human milk.[19] It is not clear if the role of cholesterol in human milk, where it is largely in the globule membrane, is nutritional and desirable, or physical and related to the process of milk fat secretion. Studies in other species have found early lipid nutrition influences cholesterol metabolism in later life.[27] The incidence of arterial lesions, and plasma low/high density lipoprotien cholesterol was higher, not lower, in non-human primates which were breast-fed rather than fed formula as infants.[27]

FATTY ACID REQUIREMENTS OF PREMATURE INFANTS

It is likely that arachidonic acid (20:4n–6) and docosahexaenoic acid (22:6n–3) are acquired by the fetus largely by placental transfer, released to the fetal circulation as unesterified fatty acids and transferred to developing organs bound to alpha-fetoprotein or in low or high denisty lipoprotein lipids.[1] If uptake of 20:4n–6 and 22:6n–3 from plasma is an important source of these fatty acids for brain growth, then maintenance of circulating lipid 20:4n–6 and 22:6n–3 at levels equivalent to those expected in utero is a reasonable goal for the lipid nutrition of premature infants. This is difficult for a number of reasons, including differences in the composition of parenteral and enteral formulas and milk from that of the free fatty acids released by the placenta, obvious metabolic effects of the different route and form of delivery, possible metabolic and hormonal changes due to increased dependence on fat rather than glucose for energy, and altered nutrient needs in the extrauterine environment.

Changes in blood lipid n-6 and n-3 fatty acids after premature birth

Blood lipid levels of 20:4n–6 and 22:6n–3 decrease rapidly following very premature birth, particularly when energy and/or lipid intakes are restricted.[1,10,19] It is not clear if the decline is due to energy deficit, resulting in oxidation of 18:2n–6 and 18:3n–3 for energy to sustain essential functions, inappropriate compositions of parenteral lipid emulsions, or low tissue desaturase activities. It is reasonable to argue that fattty acid compositional development in the CNS should be sustained equivalent to that in utero, irrespective of whether energy requirements can be met or whether nutritional support is from parenteral or enteral solutions. Unlike 18:2n–6 and 18:3n–3, 20:4n–6 and 22:6n–3 are preferentially incorporated into phospholipids. These considerations provide a reasonable argument to advocate that a source of preformed 20:4n–6 and 22:6n–3 is provided to premature infants from birth.

Blood lipid levels of 20:4n–6 and 22:6n–3 are lower in premature infants fed formula with 18:2n–6 and 18:3n–3 as the only n-6 and n-3 fatty acids than in infants fed expressed human milk. Although 20:4n–6 and 22:6n–3 levels stabilize in premature infants receiving full-volume feedings with expressed milk, levels are not restored to those expected in utero or in breast-fed term infants.[1,10] Whether this reflects increased requirements to replenish tissue stores or support rapid growth, and thus requirements in excess of that provided by human milk, is not known. However, it seems that irrespective of feeding with human milk, small premature infants have low blood 20:4n–6 and 22:6n–3; the degree of depletion seems related to the length of parental nutrition and time to regain birth weight, and with this, the degree of prematurity.

Effect of formula n-6 and n-3 fatty acids on growth and CNS development in premature infants

Blood lipid 20:4n–6 and 22:6n–3 can be increased in premature infants by feeding formulas with oils containing 20:4n–6 and 22:6n–3.[28-31] Electroretinograph recordings found lower rod, but not cone function at 36 weeks postconception in infants fed formula with 0.25% kcal linolenic acid (18:3n–3) than in infants fed human milk.[28] This amount of 18:3n–3 is below that needed to support maximum retina and synaptic membrane docosahexaenoic acid in term gestation animals,[10] and below the intake recommended by the European Society for Paediatric Gastroenterology and Nutrition[32] and for infant diets in Canada.[1,19] Electroretinograph recordings were not different between premature infants fed formula with about 1.3% kcal (2.7% fatty acids) 18:3n–3 and infants fed human milk, and no differences were found among any of the infants at 57 weeks post-conception.[28] In other studies, infants fed formula with 22:6n–3 from fish oil showed higher visual acuity in Teller acuity card tests at 48 and 57 weeks postconception, but not thereafter, than infants fed a similar formula with 1% kcal 18:3n–3 and no fish oil.[29] Normalized body weight, head circumference and length gains, and performance in tests of cognitive, psychomotor and mental development, however, were lower in infants fed the formula with fish oil; these differences did not become statistically apparent until 79–93 weeks postconception.[29,33] The further decrease in 20:4n–6 caused by feeding formula with fish oil is probably explained by inhibition of desaturation of 18:2n–6 to 20:4n–6, and competition from 20:5n–3 for incorporation into phospholipids.[1] A statistical relationship was found between growth and 20:4n–6,[33] but evidence to support a direct causal relationship between 20:4n–6 and growth, mental or psychomotor development is not available. Plasma 20:4n–6 is lower in term infants fed formula rather than human milk, but growth is not slower.[1,34] There are no published data to demonstrate addition of 20:4n–6 to formulas will prevent the adverse effects of fish oil, or to show safety of 20:4n–6 or 22:6n–3 from any source other than human milk.

MEDIUM CHAIN TRIGLYCERIDES

The clinical usefulness of MCT rests on greater solubility of medium chain fatty acids in water than of long chain fatty acids.[19,25] MCT can also be absorbed intact, and require lower bile acid and colipase-dependent pancreatic lipase concentrations for micelle formation and hydrolysis than needed for triglycerides with long chain fatty acids. The bile salt pool, intraluminal bile salt concentrations and colipase-dependent lipase activity is often low in small preterm infants.[19]

Medium chain fatty acid transport and tissue storage

Once absorbed, medium chain fatty acids are transported predominantly as unesterified fatty acids through the portal vein to the liver. Transfer into the mitochondria is independent of the carnitine acyl-transferase system, and beta-oxidation to acetyl coenzyme A is rapid. The activity of acyl transferases with medium chain fatty acid substrates is low. It is not surprising, therefore, that tissue levels of 8:0, 10:0 and 12:0 remain very low, even in premature infants fed formulas with 40–50% medium chain fatty acid.[35] Lauric acid (14:0) is partly transported in chylomicron triglycerides and acylated; the amounts in infant adipose tissues increase in relation to the amount in the formula.[35] The lower plasma 20:4n–6 and 22:6n–3 associated with formula feeding also seems to be exacerbated when MCT rather than palmitic acid (16:0) is used as the source of saturated fatty acids in formula fed to piglets.[36] The significance of this to interpretations of n-6 and n-3 fatty acid requirements from studies on premature infants fed formulas with high amounts of MCT is not clear.

Medium chain fatty acid oxidation

Despite arguments that MCT confer advantages to fat absorption, several recent studies have found no difference in weight gain, head circumference or linear growth of premature infants fed formula with MCT rather than long chain fatty acids.[37–39] Although rapidly oxidized to acetyl coenzyme A, only 32–64% MCT fed to premature infants was oxidized completely to carbon dioxide[40] The remaining acetyl coenzyme A produced by oxidation of the medium chain fatty acids is presumably used for de novo synthesis of palmitic acid (16:0). The energy wastage associated with fat oxidation then biosynthesis, compared to direct incorporation of dietary long chain fatty acids into tissues, may explain the absence of improved energy or weight gain in infants fed MCT.

Plasma ketone and urinary dicarboxylic acid concentrations, primarily adipic (C6), suberic (C8) and sebacic (C10) acid, increase in premature infants in relation to the amount of MCT in the formula.[19] Ketone bodies are formed by condensation of acetyl coenzyme A when the rate of acetyl coenzyme A production (from fatty acid oxidation) exceeds the capacity for further oxidation via the tricarboxylic acid cycle.[19] Dicarboxylic acids are the products of fatty acid omega-oxidation involving cytochrome P450 of the endoplasmic reticulum and cytosolic dehydrogenase. Urinary concentrations of sebacic acid 200-fold above normal have been reported for infants fed formula with 40% fat from MCT.[19] The amount of energy lost to the urine, however, is less than 1–2%. Giving MCT to generate ketone bodies to provide energy, or substrates for synthesis of cholesterol and fatty acids, in brain should not be necessary in appropriately fed premature infants.[28] Although MCT in formula should not be replaced by fats which compromise fat or mineral absorption, pathways of fatty acid metabolism are unlikely to resemble that of infants fed human milk if formulas containing significant amounts of MCT are fed.

KEY POINTS FOR CLINICAL PRACTICE

- Recommendations for the fatty acid composition of infant formulas have generally been based on the composition of human milk rather than direct information on infant fatty acid requirements. It is reasonable to assume that, as for other nutrients, the fat content and range of fatty acids in human milk cover the needs of healthy, term newborns.

- Arachidonic acid (20:4n-6) and docosahexaenoic acid (22:6n-3) are not essential dietary nutrients for the term newborn of other species. If maximum tissue phospholipid 20:4n-6 and 22:6n-3 are used as the criteria from which to establish dietary requirements, then the minimum requirement for linoleic (18:2n-6) and linolenic (18:3n-3) acid in other species is 3% and 0.7% kcal respectively.

- Human milk cannot be used as the standard on which to base suitable upper limits, or ratios for 18:2n-6 and 18:3n-3 because human milk contains 20:4n-6 and 22:6n-3. Ratios of 18:2n-6/18: 3n-3 of 4:1 to 16:1 seem to be compatible with maximum tissue levels of 20:4n-6 and 22: 6n-3.

- The major concern regarding 20:4n-6 and 22:6n-3 is the supply to the CNS. The requirements for these fatty acids may, therefore, be best related to the rate and stage of brain growth. The supply of 20:4n-6 and 22:6n-3 to the CNS should not be limited by the ability to provide premature infants with full-volume enteral feeds of formulas or milk.

- The increased rate of development of visual acuity observed in premature infants fed formulas with 22:6n-3 seems to be transient, and formula with fish oils can reduce growth, psychomotor and mental development. Scientific knowledge does not permit a conclusion that the growth and developmental problems experienced by premature infants fed formulas with fish oil were caused by 20:5n-3 in the oil, or due to a lack of 20:4n-6 in the formula.

- Studies of long-term development of infants fed 20:4n-6 from sources other than human milk, or fed 22:6n-3 from oils other then fish oil, have not beeen reported. It is prudent, therefore, to advocate the use of expressed human milk as the most appropriate source of fatty acid nutrition for premature infants.

REFERENCES

1 Innis SM. Essential fatty acids in growth and development. Prog Lipid Res 1991; 30: 39–103
2 Innis SM. Human milk and formula fatty acids. J Pediatr 1992; 120: S56–S61
3 Jensen RG. In: Lebenthal E, ed. Lipids in human milk: composition and fat-soluble vitamins. Textbook of gastroenterology and nutrition in infancy. 2nd ed. New York: Raven Press 1989: pp 157–208
4 Fliesler SJ, Anderson RE. Chemistry and metabolism of lipids in the vertebrate retina. Prog Lipid Res 1983; 22: 77–131
5 Sastry PS. Lipids of nervous tissue: composition and metabolism. Prog Lipid Res 1985; 24: 69–176

6 Martinez M. Tissue levels of polyunsaturated fatty acids during early human development J Pediatr 1992; 120: S129–S138

7 Moore SA, Yoder E, Murphy S et al. Astrocytes, not neurons, produce docosahexaenoic acid (22:ω-6) and arachidonic acid (20:4ω-6). J Neurochem 1991; 56: 518–524

8 Voss A, Reinhart M, Sprecher H. Differences in the interconversion between 20- and 22-carbon (n-3) and (n-6) polyunsaturated fatty acids in rat liver. Biochim Biophys Acta 1992; 1127: 33–40

9 Bourre J-M, Francois M, Youyou A G et al. The effects of dietary α-linolenic acid on the composition of nerve membranes, enzymatic activity, amplitude of electrophysiological parameters, resistance to poisons and performance of learning tasks in rats. J Nutr 1989; 119: 1880–1892

10 Innis SM. N-3 fatty acid requirements of the newborn. Lipids 1992; 27: 879–885

11 Innis SM. Plasma and red blood cell fatty acid values as indexes of essential fatty acids in the developing organs of infants fed with milk or formulas. J Pediatr 1992; 120: S78–S86

12 Arnold J, Leslie G, Chen S. Protein, lactose and fat concentration of breast milk of mothers of term and premature neonates. Aust Paediatr J 1987; 23: 299–300

13 Lepage G, Collet S, Bougle D et al. The composition of preterm milk in relation to the degree of prematurity. Am J Clin Nutr 1984; 40: 1042–1049

14 Silber GH, Hachey DL, Schanler RF et al. Manipulation of maternal diet to alter fatty acid composition of human milk intended for premature infants. Am J Clin Nutr 1988; 47: 810–814

15 Harzer G, Dieterich I, Haug M. Effects of the diet on the composition of human milk. Ann Nutr Metab 1984; 28: 231–239

16 Clark RM, Hundrieser KE. Changes in cholesterol esters of human milk with total milk lipid. J Pediatr Gastroenterol Nutr 1989; 9: 347–350

17 Potter JM, Nestel PJ. The effects of dietary fatty acids and cholesterol on the milk lipids of lactating women and the plasma cholesterol of breast-fed infants. Am J Clin Nutr 1976; 29: 54–60

18 Koletzko B. Zurfur, Stoffwechsel und biologische Wirkungen transisomerer Fettsauren bei Säuglingen. Nahrung 1991; 35: 229–283

19 Innis SM. Nutritional needs of the preterm infant: fat. In: Tsang RC, Lucas A, Mally R, Ziotkin S, eds. Nutrition in infancy. 2nd edn. Caudicus Medical Pawling, NY 1992

20 Sanders TAB, Reddy S. The influence of a vegetarian diet on the fatty acid composition of human milk and the essential fatty acid status of the infant. J Pediatr 1992; 120: S71–S77

21 Hamosh M. Lipid metabolism in premature infants. Biol Neonate 1987; 52: 50–64

22 Hernell O, Blackberg L, Bernback S. Digestion of human milk fat in early infancy. Acta Paediatr Scand Suppl 1989; 351: 57–62

23 Filer LJ, Mattson FH, Foman SJ. Triglyceride configuration and fat absorption by the human infant. J Nutr 1969; 99: 293–298

24 Jensen C, Buist NRM, Wilson T. Absorption of individual fatty acids from long chain or medium chain triglycerides in very small infants. Am J Clin Nutr 1986; 43: 745–751

25 Bach AC, Babayan V. Medium-chain triglycerides: an update. Am J Clin Nutr 1982; 36: 950–962

26 Chappell JE, Clandinin MT, Kearney-Volpe C et al. Fatty acid balance studies in premature infants fed human milk or formula: effect of calcium supplementation. J Pediatr 1986; 108: 439–447

27 Lewis DS, Mott GE, McMahan CA et al. Deferred effects of preweaning diet on atherosclerosis in adolescent baboons. Arteriosclerosis 1989; 8: 274–280

28 Birch DG, Birch EE, Hoffman DR et al. Retinal development in very low-birth-weight infants fed diets differing in omega-3 fatty acids. Invest Ophthalmol 1992; Vis Sci 33: 2365–2376

29 Carlson SE, Cooke RJ, Rhodes PG et al. Effect of vegetable and marine oils in preterm infant formulas on blood arachidonic and docosahexaenoic acids. J Pediatr 120: S159–S167

30 Clandinin MT, Parrot A, Van Aerde JE et al. Feeding preterm infants a formula containing C20 and C22 fatty acids stimulates plasma phospholipid fatty acid composition of infants fed human milk. Early Hum Dev 1992; 31: 41–51

31 Koletzko B, Schmidt E, Bremer HJ et al. Effects of dietary long-chain polyunsaturated fatty acids on the essential fatty acid status of premature infants. Eur J Pediatr 1989; 148: 669–675

32 ESPGAN Committee on Nutrition. Comment on the content and composition of lipids in infant formula. Acta Paediatr Scand 1991; 80: 887–896

33 Carlson SE, Cooke RJ, Werkman SH et al. First year growth of preterm infants fed standard compared to marine-oil n-3 supplemented formula. Lipids 1992; 27: 901–907

34 Dewey KG, Hening MJ, Nommsen LA et al. Growth of breast-fed and formula-fed infants from 0 to 18 months: the DARLING study. Pediatrics 1992; 89: 1035–1041

35 Sarda P, Lepage G, Roy CC et al. Storage of medium-chain triglycerides in adipose tissue of orally fed infants. Am J Clin Nutr 1987; 45: 399–405

36 Wall KM, Diersen-Schade D, Innis SM. Nonessential fatty acids in formula fat blends influence essential fatty acid metabolism and composition in plasma and organ lipid classes. Lipids 1992; 27: 1024–1031

37 Bustamante SA, Fiello A, Pollack PF. Growth of premature infants fed formulas with 10%, 30% or 50% medium-chain triglycerides. Am J Dis Child 1987; 141: 516–519

38 Hamosh M, Mehta NR, Fink CS et al. Fat absorption in premature infants: medium-chain trigylcerides and long-chain triglycerides are absorbed from formula at similar rates. J Pediatr Gastroenterol Nutr 1991; 13: 143–149

39 Whyte RK, Campbell D, Stanhope R et al. Energy balance in low birth-weight infants fed formula of high or low medium-chain triglyceride content. J Pediatr 1986; 108: 964–971

40 Sulkers EJ, Lafeberm HN, Sauer PJJ. Quantitation of oxidation of medium chain triglycerides in preterm infants. Pediatr Res 1989; 26: 294–297

12

Communication disorders

L. Rosenbloom

Defining developmental disorders, including those of children's language, produces a number of difficulties. These include the need to recognize that there must inevitably be a continuum between normal and abnormal development and that any cut-off will be arbitrary and at best statistically or clinically rather than pathologically based. Secondly, and because child development is a dynamic process, what is within the normal range at a young age will not be necessarily so for older children. Thirdly, and this applies particularly to child language, environmental considerations are a very major determinant of function and require evaluation in their own right.

Against this background, communication disorders in childhood pose clinically important problems and aspects of their epidemiology, classification, causes and associations, treatment and outcomes will be presented and discussed.

EPIDEMIOLOGY

Mac Keith and Rutter[1] concluded on the basis of their literature review that 1% of children came to school with a marked language handicap and that a further 4–5% may also show the sequelae of earlier language difficulties. The early studies reviewed by these authors and others[2] tended to rely on estimates of speech and expressive language rather than on verbal comprehension which is more difficult to assess clinically. However, since standardized language tests have become available,[3] more detailed breakdowns of specific populations have been performed and have proved helpful, both in estimating the overall prevalence of speech and language problems and also on how they break down into specific disorders. Among the most useful of these has been the Dunedin Multidisciplinary Health and Development Study[4] in which more than 1000 3-year-olds were examined. Language delay was defined as a score at or below the fifth centile in verbal comprehension, verbal expression or both. In all, 7.6% of the population was identified as language-delayed, with approximately a third of these having comprehension problems only, a third having expressive problems and a third both.

The longitudinal significance of preschool language delay has been reviewed and summarized by Silva.[5] He concluded that it is not clear whether early language delay truly predicts the later development of specific and severe language disorders. Given that there is a general consensus that around 1% of children have a severe and established language delay, resolution of their problems must occur for the majority of preschoolers with speech and language difficulties.

However, in studies from both the UK[6,7] and New Zealand,[4] a clear association is demonstrated between early language delay and later measured intelligence and reading difficulties. In addition, the British studies showed a high degree of later behavioural disturbance for their children on follow-up.

These findings beg a number of questions with respect to the value of surveillance and early intervention programmes for children who present with language delay. These are likely to have only a limited value if the prevention and treatment of specific language disorders are their principal criteria, but may be more useful in a wider developmental context.

Other population studies on children with language disorders have focused upon specific groups or specific problems and provide valuable cross-sectional and outcome data. Thus, Robinson,[8] in a detailed examination of children attending a residential school, demonstrated the range of associated factors and problems that accompany so-called specific language disorders, whilst Lotter[9] summarized the poor prognosis for autistic children as they progress into adult life.

CLASSIFICATION

Historically, classification of speech and language disorders has had a medical basis,[10] but in many ways this is unsatisfactory as labels and descriptions fail to distinguish between clinical features, their presumed causation and, when it is known, their pathogenesis. This situation is analogous to that for cerebral palsy.

One reaction has been to reject medically oriented classifications and instead to describe children in terms of their linguistic criteria, so that the different components of language and their qualities are described. These are shown in Table 12.1.

Bishop & Rosenbloom[11] have correlated the medical and linguistic approaches to classification by taking as their starting point particular varieties of language abnormality, and then describing the medical and other factors that underlie them when these are known. A modification of their classification is given in Table 12.2.

Within the paediatric context, a number of the disorders identified in Table 12.2 and their associated factors merit more detailed consideration.

THE CAUSES OF LANGUAGE DISORDERS

Prenatal and perinatal determinants

Given that so many of the neurological disorders that cause childhood handicap are prenatally determined, either before conception as genetically

Table 12.1   The components of language

Component	Definition	Examples of abnormality
Phonology	Sound system	Consonant or syllable deletion or substitution
Grammar	Structure of language	Telegrammatic sentence structure
	Syntax and morphology	Incorrect generalization of grammatical rules
Semantics	Representation of meaning	Vocabulary confusion Incorrect generalization of meanings of words or phrases
Pragmatics	How language is used	Misunderstanding of social components of communication

Table 12.2   Classification of language disorders

1 Speech limited in quality and/or quantity but other language skills normal
   (a) Structural or sensorimotor defects or speech
      apparatus producing dysphonia or dysarthria
   (b) Deafness acquired after language has developed
   (c) Elective mutism
   (d) Dysfluency

2. Generalized delay of language development
   (a) Common with most types of mental handicap
   (b) Environmental deprivation
   (c) ? Consequence of chronic conductive hearing loss
   (d) Idiopathic, possible a developmental variant

3. Specific problems with phonology and syntax
   (a) Phonological syntactic syndrome
   (b) Left hemisphere lesions in older children
   (c) ? Consequence of high-frequency hearing loss

4. Specific problems with semantics and pragmatics
   (a) Semantic-pragmatic disorder
   (b) Mild autism   } ? The same
   (c) Asperger's syndrome   }   condition
   (d) Cocktail-party syndrome[12] }

5. Poor understanding and limited expression
   (a) Severe mental handicap
   (b) Severe/profound prelingual deafness
   (c) Acquired bilateral lesions of language areas (Landau–Kleffner syndrome)
   (d) Congenital auditory imperception

6. Severe impairment of non-verbal and verbal communication
   (a) Severe/profound mental handicap
   (b) Infantile autism
   (c) Ultimate outcome of degenerative disorders

produced characteristics or subsequent to conception during the processes of central nervous system formation and maturation, and given the recognized preponderance of boys with language disorders, it is perhaps surprising that the association between prenatal factors and language impairment as the specific or dominating clinical feature has been of relatively recent interest. However, Mutton & Lea[13] demonstrated an increased incidence of the order of 3.5 of an assortment of chromosomal defects in language-disordered children, whilst follow-up studies of infants found on newborn screening to have sex chromosome abnormalities showed that many have delayed language development and speech problems.[14] This was most often, albeit inconsistently, demonstrated in boys with Klinefelter syndrome (XXY). The fragile X syndrome is also reported to have an association with language disorders including infantile autism, but a recent review[15] makes it clear that the behavioural phenotype of this syndrome can be very wide indeed.

Other non-chromosomal abnormalities of prenatal origin, e.g. galactosaemia,[16] Williams syndrome (infantile hypercalcaemia) and Sotos syndrome (cerebral gigantism) are recognized to have language problems as part of their phenotype, whilst the recognized familial incidence of autism[17] indicates the probability of a genetic contribution to that disorder.

It is not surprising therefore that in clinical practice it is very common indeed to obtain a positive family history for language disorders,[8] and this should always be sought.

By contrast, there is a very weak association indeed between perinatal risk factors and specific language disorders. The hazards of prematurity, hypoxia, trauma and infection are all more likely to produce either generalized brain damage with very widespread functional impairment or specific evidence of cerebral palsy with accompanying motor dysfunction. It is presumed that the plasticity of the central nervous system at this time is such that the discrete areas of left hemispheric damage that would need to be the basis of specific language impairments have their function taken over by the opposite hemisphere. Goodman[18] has discussed the relationship of perinatal problems to autism and has concluded that, as for other language disorders, there is no convincing evidence that autism is a consequence rather than a cause of perinatal complications.

The significance of hearing loss

When acquired after language has fully developed, hearing loss has little effect on verbal skills but it does interfere with understanding spoken language and causes a deterioration in articulation and voice quality. By contrast, prelingual deafness has profound consequences for language development even with early diagnosis and amplification, with the most striking characteristics being an inflexible use of vocabulary and limited sentence structures. These problems extend to written and signed language also.

It is also often assumed that 'deaf speech' is easily recognized, but while this may be true for children with a severe hearing loss, it is not the case for those with milder losses or those affecting higher frequencies. It is not only this author's experience that the single most common error in investigating a child who fails to develop language is to overlook a peripheral hearing loss.

Conductive hearing loss, primarily due to glue ear and which may therefore be intermittent, is more likely to be a risk factor for language development than a specific cause of disordered language. This subject was well-reviewed by Paradise[19] and Hall & Hill,[20] all of whom make the point that, given a combination of appropriate treatment and teaching, the majority of children do not suffer adverse developmental sequelae to conductive hearing loss. However, a minority will, with perhaps listening and memory skills being particularly adversely affected.

Environmental influences

Exposure of a child to language is necessary for the child's own language to develop and it is reasonable to extrapolate from this to suggest that lesser degrees of environmental deprivation will impair language development to some degree. When reviewing this subject, Puckering & Rutter[21] make the points that, within the normal range of environments, rearing in a socially disadvantaged home, being one of a pair of twins, being brought up in a very large family, and having parents who play and talk little may retard language development. By contrast, rearing in a family that provides rich and varied interactions and responses, and reciprocal conversation may accelerate language development. These differences will lead to variations in the rates that children acquire language and may well have a significance for their later scholastic achievements.

Specific attention has also been paid to the effects of abuse and neglect on the development of speech and language,[22] and it is probable that problems in these areas are the commonest developmental sequelae of child abuse. Both expressive language and verbal comprehension are affected. Included among the reasons for this are that language may be more sensitive to environmental influences than other aspects of cognition and that the majority of abused children are boys under the age of 5 years and hence are particularly vulnerable.

The significance of these studies is the implication that appropriate remedial attention may reverse the effects of adverse environmental influences on language development, although hitherto there has been no reported controlled study of intervention to promote communication skills of abused or neglected children.

Developmental speech and language disorders

Many children present with a language disorder for which there is no obvious explanation. Peripheral hearing is normal, non-verbal intelligence is good, the environment is appropriate and there are no signs of physical or psychiatric abnormality even after detailed investigation.

This grouping includes a large number of children who will in due course, and in retrospect, be demonstrated merely to have had delayed language development. The epidemiological and environmental studies referred to earlier in this chapter make it clear that the language delay seen in many very young children will resolve either spontaneously or with help, with or without non-linguistic long-term sequelae. However, a minority do not so resolve and their specific language difficulties remain.

It is logical under these circumstances to assume that neurological maturation has in some specific structural or functional way gone awry and the description of 'developmental' for these children's problems is appropriate. Support for this hypothesis comes firstly from what is envisaged to be the normal way in which language is acquired. This assumes that infants have an innate language acquisition mechanism[23] which enables them to formulate relevant rules for learning and that on occasion this must function imperfectly. Secondly, and as is described presently, detailed examination and investigation of children with specific developmental language disorders not infrequently demonstrate subtle evidence of other neurological abnormalities, e.g. clumsiness and perceptual difficulties.

CLINICAL FEATURES OF COMMUNICATION DISORDERS

A degree of selection is inevitable in this section and disorders which have a particular interest or relevance for paediatric practice are primarily considered.

Phonological syntactic disorder

This is the most common variety of developmental language disorder in which apparently normal children have selective difficulties with language structure and form, but have normal language content. Thus, they have a normal urge to communicate and say sensible and appropriate things, but have difficulties with both phonology and syntax. There is a wide range of severity, with at one extreme children who would traditionally be referred to as having developmental expressive aphasia with unintelligible speech and syntactic structures several years behind their age level. At the other extreme are children whose main problems are with phonology and who would in the past have been regarded as having functional articulation problems. Boys are much more frequently affected than girls.

Parents typically report that language development was slow from birth. A positive family history of language or reading difficulties is common. Language does improve slowly, preferably with the assistance of much individual and small-group work, but the children usually have difficulty learning to read and are often far behind in basic school attainments and social development by the time that reasonable expressive speech is acquired.

Although problems with expressive language dominate the clinical picture, affected individuals may also be demonstrated to have other evidence of oromotor dysfunction[24] with difficulties in sucking, swallowing or chewing, to be clumsy or have perceptual difficulties,[25] or to have additional receptive language difficulties.[26] These emphasize the requirement that is presently discussed for children who present in this way to have multidisciplinary assessment and investigation.

Developmental receptive disorders

This comprises a heterogeneous collection of problems. At the severe extreme is the rare condition variously described as congenital auditory imperception or developmental receptive aphasia. So far as can be determined, hearing is normal, although many have postulated the existence of a central, i.e. cerebral, auditory deficit. There is virtually a total absence of verbal understanding and an accompanying absence of speech. Clinically, the situation is analogous to the more severe examples of Landau–Kleffner syndrome (acquired aphasia with epilepsy) with preservation of non-verbal and social skills at least initially. It is extremely uncommon, and the author has seen only 2 children who fulfilled the diagnostic criteria, 1 of whom has been the subject of a case report.[27] In the long term, the language difficulties of both children resolved without overt educational or social sequelae.

Inevitably, many children who are considered to have developmental receptive aphasia turn out to have an undiagnosed hearing loss and scrupulous and repeated audiological investigation is mandatory if this condition is suspected.

Much more commonly seen are children who have a combination of some degree of impairment of receptive and expressive abilities, not infrequently seen against a background of a lesser degree of impairment of cognitive skills generally. These form the bulk of language clinic referrals[28] and their evaluation and treatment require a combination of audiological, paediatric, psychological and speech and language therapy expertise. They require to be distinguished from other varieties of language disorder, children who have generalized or specific learning difficulties that are not primarily linguistic and those who have primary attentional or behavioural problems.

A small proportion of language-disordered children have auditory memory or word-finding difficulties that are demonstrable on psycholinguistic testing. They are sometimes accompanied by electroencephalographic dysrhythmias localized to the left temporal or both temporal regions. Even in the absence of a frank seizure disorder, a trial of anticonvulsant therapy may be indicated in these children. In the author's practice this has sometimes proved beneficial, although hitherto there are no reported studies of this approach.

Acquired language disorders

When previously demonstrable linguistic skills are lost, there is always cause for concern. Acquired hearing loss has already been considered and regression of speech and language may also be seen following head injuries, in adverse environmental circumstances, including child abuse and neglect, and as a component of any chronic and debilitating childhood illness.

More specifically, a deterioration in language may be part of the generalized regression that is seen in the whole range of degenerative neurological disorders and indeed may be the index feature of these. In such circumstances, careful clinical and investigational evaluation should indicate the nature of the child's disorder, preferably sooner rather than later, although this is not always the case.[29]

In addition to these general considerations, three particular conditions merit more detailed description: acquired aphasia with epilepsy, elective mutism, and disintegrative psychosis.

Acquired aphasia with epilepsy

Landau & Kleffner[30] described this condition, which is eponymously linked with them. Typically, a previously normal child loses language skills between the ages of 3 and 9, without other neurological abnormalities or known brain pathology. Both receptive and expressive abilities are lost, sometimes acutely, and the child may be thought to be deaf. The loss of the ability to communicate may lead to severe behavioural disturbance. At much the same time most, but not all, affected children develop generalized or partial seizures, but all have dysrhythmic electroencephalograms with bilateral but asymmetrical paroxysmal discharges mainly over the postcentral and temporal areas.

The course of the disease is very variable, with some of the affected children having a severe language disorder, usually with accompanying epilepsy, that persists into adult life. Others recover quickly and completely whilst a few have recurrent aphasic episodes sometimes heralded by an exacerbation of seizure activity. Gordon[31] has suggested that the primary disorder in affected children is a disruption of cerebral function by epileptic activity and this is possibly consistent with the observation of Bishop[32] that the older the age of onset, the better is the long-term prognosis.

Treatment with anticonvulsants is appropriate but of variable benefit. Other measures that have been tried include corticosteroids and neurosurgical subpial resection.

Elective mutism

This term is used to describe children who are known to be able to talk, but refuse to speak in all but a few situations and appear to be excessively shy. It may be necessary to observe through a one-way screen the child with a parent or use previously obtained recordings in order to acquire a language sample. It is important to appreciate that a significant proportion of electively mute children do have articulatory or language deficits. In such cases, reticence may be an understandable reaction to the experience of being teased, criticized or not understood.

Others can speak normally but fail to do so. They do not have a language disorder, but are likely to show other features of childhood psychiatric disorder. Conversely, the absence of these additional features of emotional disturbance makes it unlikely that mutism is the presentation of a psychiatric disturbance.

Disintegrative psychosis

The clinical characteristics of this rare and probably inappropriately named condition were detailed by Evans-Jones & Rosenbloom.[33] Typically, children who have developed normal language and other skills then rapidly lose these abilities between 3 and 5 years of age. This is often at a time of severe psychological stress which may well be a precipitating factor. Over a period of weeks or months affected children lose their psychosocial skills, although motor abilities are not affected, and become severely retarded and autistic. No specific aetiology has been demonstrated in these children who, on prolonged follow-up, remain profoundly handicapped and occasionally epileptic, but do not show further deterioration.

Autism and related disorders

It is now 50 years since Kanner first described early childhood autism[34] and controversy and confusion persist with regard to the clinical features that merit the use of this diagnostic label, its pathogenesis, the implications for development of affected individuals and its relationship to other disorders, including Asperger's syndrome, semantic-pragmatic disorder and pervasive developmental disorder.

The diagnosis of autism is based on three main criteria:
1. Delayed and deviant language development, which is out of keeping with the child's non-verbal development and which affects non-verbal and abstract skills as well as spoken language.
2. Delayed and deviant social development, which again is out of keeping with the child's development in other areas.
3. The presence of obsessional rituals and routines and general resistance to change.

Despite the fact that all autistic children exhibit the core symptoms of language deficits, social impairments and resistance to change, the extent of their handicap can vary widely. The cognitive impairment ranges from moderate or severe retardation in more than half, to normal performance on non-verbal tasks in 20%. The language handicap ranges from children who remain non-communicating and severely limited in their receptive language skills to those who show only mild developmental delays and whose acquisition of syntax is relatively good. The overwhelming deficit in this latter group is their deviant use of language for communiction. Social abnormalities range from almost total withdrawal from social contact to indiscriminate approaches to complete strangers.

The extent of rituals and routines also varies, with differences often being related to levels of intelligence. In more severely retarded individuals, the main feature tends to be their stereotyped repetitive use of objects e.g. spinning or flicking. In more intelligent autistic children, the obsessions may be extremely complex and pervasive and tend to involve other people as well as themselves.

Thus, there is a very varied clinical picture which is made more complicated by the fact that patterns of skills and handicaps change with age and this has led to a search for greater refinement in diagnosis and classification.

The American classification of DSM-III[35] represents an attempt to differentiate between children within the autistic spectrum and has generated the label of pervasive developmental disorder together with a variety of subcategories. However, this has not proved popular in clinical practice in the UK or Europe, and the validity of the subgroupings has been a source of contention.[36]

Clinical practice has probably not been much helped either by a proliferation of labels that may or may not be associated with autism, but two of these — Asperger's syndrome and semantic-pragmatic disorder — require more detailed consideration because of their relatively widespread usage.

Asperger's original description in German in 1944[37] is essentially of a mild form of autism distinct from that described by Kanner, but several authors, notably Wing[38] and Bowman,[39] have coherently argued that they are a continuum but that Asperger's syndrome is a useful term to explain the problems of autistic adults and children who do not show mutism or severe withdrawal but nevertheless have impaired social interaction and very circumscribed interests.

The term semantic-pragmatic syndrome was first introduced by Rapin & Allen[24] to describe a group of children who use superficially complex language with clear articulation, but whose use and understanding of language, especially in social communication, are defective. Although Rapin & Allen considered that this inability to use language appropriately in a social context could be distinguished in many cases from autism, this has not been this author's experience[11] or that of Bishop.[11,40] It would seem appropriate therefore to regard semantic and pragmatic linguistic difficulties in childhood as indicating the presence of a disorder which is at the mild end of the autistic continuum and hence may not overtly be associated with deviant social development and obsessional characteristics.

It is now generally accepted that autism has its basis in organic brain disease, but it is not possible to be more precise than this. Epilepsy is seen eventually in up to a third of autistic people, but neurological investigations have not demonstrated any consistent abnormalities. Similarly, a genetic contribution is also accepted, but the modes of inheritance are unclear, as also are the genetic links with other learning disorders which are often seen in the families of autistic children. It is also of clinical concern that there appears to have been a recent significant increase in the numbers of autistic children presenting to paediatric services. The cause of this is unknown, but is not related to the sequelae of perinatal adversity.

In spite of many false dawns, there is no replicated research evidence that a variety of drug treatments, including fenfluramine, vitamin or hormone therapy or behavioural approaches, including holding therapy, significantly influence or benefit autistic symptomatology for the majority of affected individuals, although occasional single case studies and anecdotes are quoted to counter this. In general, however, the most promising practical approach to treatment seems to be the provision of appropriate and structured educational facilities from an early age and the availability of behaviourally based counselling for parents at home.[41] It is important to control the social and cognitive demands made on autistic children and help them to make the best of their existing skills.

Nevertheless, the prognosis for independence is poor, and although a small minority of autistic children who have good intelligence and develop language are able ultimately to leave home, obtain employment and occasionally marry, their social skills usually remain overtly limited.

KEY POINTS FOR CLINICAL PRACTICE

- Communication disorders are usually an expression of neurological dysfunction and hence require a similar clinical approach to other neurological disorders. In practice, this entails a full personal, developmental and family history followed by audiological, developmental and neurological examinations. These form the basis for more detailed psycholinguistic evaluation. The methodology and practical application of this team approach in the author's department have been described by Neville and Gunn.[42]
- The yield from investigating language-disordered children is poor. Nevertheless, it is legitimate to ask for chromosome studies and to have a low threshold for performing some biochemical investigations, including amino acid chromatography. Further biochemical, neurophysiological and imaging studies may be indicated, e.g. in the presence of focal abnormal neurology, hearing loss, epilepsy or unexpected features such as memory difficulties on detailed psycholinguistic testing. The criterion to be applied

is whether the investigation results, whether normal or abnormal, are likely to affect management.

- Follow-up and periodic re-evaluation are mandatory. There is a very wide range of potential outcomes. Those for whom delayed language is a developmental variant may well 'grow out of it' but are nevertheless socially and educationally vulnerable at a very sensitive time in their lives. Similarly, hearing loss is potentially recognizable and treatable, although this is not always achieved in practice. Even when it is, there are major implications for linguistic and social development.

- One major implication of early language delay is that many affected children will subsequently be demonstrated to have more global learning difficulties and to be mentally handicapped. The recognition of this likely outcome, its appropriate investigation and the provision of genetic and other advice to the parents, together with appropriate help for the child, are legitimate components of paediatric practice. So also is the evaluation and amelioration of adverse environmental influences. Within this context it is not uncommon for child abuse and neglect to be manifested as a language disorder and sensitive investigation of family functioning and relationships is a further requirement of the paediatric and multidisciplinary approach.

- It will be readily appreciated that established and 'pure' communication disorders, even when the autistic grouping are included, are but one component of the yield from children who present with language difficulties. They are nevertheless important in their own right. Their recognition and delineation involve skilled paediatric, speech and language therapy and psychological assessments; they imply the need for appropriate parental counselling and occasionally for specific medical treatments; and they impose a requirement on educational, therapy and community child health services for the provision of relevantly staffed and skilled resources.

REFERENCES

1 Mac Keith RC, Rutter M. A note on the prevalence of speech and language disorders. In: Rutter M, Martin JAM, eds. The child with delayed speech. Clinics in developmental medicine no 43. London: SIMP with Heinemann. 1972
2 Marge M. The general problems of language disabilities in children. In: Irwin JW, Marge M, eds. Principles of childhood language disabilities. New York: Appleton Century Crofts. 1972: pp 75–98
3 Yule W. Psychologial assessment. In: Yule W, Rutter M, eds. Language development and disorders. Clinics in developmental medicine nos 101/102. Oxford: Mac Keith Press with Blackwell, 1987: pp 312–323.
4 Silva PA, Williams SM. Developmental language delay from three to seven years and its significance for low intelligence and reading difficulties at age seven. Dev Med Child Neurol 1983; 25: 783–793.
5 Silva PA. Epidemiology, longitudinal course and some associated factors. In: Yule W, Rutter M, eds. Language development and disorders. Clinics in developmental medicine nos 101/102. Oxford: Mac Keith Press with Blackwell, 1987: pp 1–15

6 Stevenson J, Richman N. The prevalence of language delay in a population of three year old children and its association with general retardation. Dev Med Child Neurol 1976; 18: 431–441

7 Fundudis T, Kolvin I, Garside RF, eds. Speech retarded and deaf children. Their psychological development. London: Academic Press. 1979

8 Robinson RJ. Causes and associations of severe and persistent specific speech and language disorders in children. Dev Med Child Neurol 1991; 33: 943–962

9 Lotter V. Follow-up studies. In: Rutter M, Schopler E, eds. Autism: a reappraisal of concepts and treatment. New York: Plenum, 1978: pp 475–495

10 Ingram TTS. The classification of speech and language disorders in young children. In: Rutter M, Martin JAM, eds. The child with delayed speech. Clinics in developmental medicine no 43. London: SIMP with Heinemann. 1972

11 Bishop DVM, Rosenbloom L. Childhood language disorders; classification and overview. In: Yule W, Rutter M, eds. Language development and disorders. Clinics in developmental medicine nos 101/102. Oxford: Mac Keith Press with Blackwell, 1987: pp 16–41

12 Hadenius AM, Hagberg B, Hytnass-Bench K, Sjogren I. The natural prognosis of infantile hydrocephalus. Acta Paediatr Scand 1962; 51: 117–118

13 Mutton DE, Lea J. Chromosome studies of children with specific speech and language delay. Dev Med Child Neurol 1980; 22: 588–594

14 Bender B, Fry E, Pennington B, Puck M, Salbenblatt J, Robinson A. Speech and language development in 41 children with sex chromosome anomalies. Pediatrics 1983; 71: 262–267

15 Goldson F, Hagerman RJ. The fragile X syndrome. Dev Med Child Neurol 1992; 34: 826–832

16 Waisbren SE, Norman TR, Schnell RR, Levy HL. Speech and language deficits in early-treated children with galactosaemia. J Pediatr 1983; 102: 75–77

17 Gilberg C, Gilberg IC, Steffenburg S. Siblings and parents of children with autism: a controlled population-based study. Dev Med Child Neurol 1992; 34: 389–398

18 Goodman R. Technical note: are perinatal complications causes or consequences of autism? J Child Psychol Psychiatry 1990; 31: 809–812

19 Paradise JL. Otitis media during early life. How hazardous to development? A critical review of the evidence. Pediatrics 1981; 68: 869–873

20 Hall DMB, Hill P. When does secretory otitis media affect language development? Arch Dis Child 1986; 61: 42–47

21 Puckering C, Rutter M. Environmental influences on language development. In: Yule W, Rutter M eds. Language development and disorders. Clinics in developmental medicine nos 101/102. Oxford: Mac Keith Press with Blackwell, 1987: pp 103–128

22 Law J, Conway J. Effect of abuse and neglect on the development of children's speech and language. Dev Med Child Neurol 1992; 34: 755–765

23 Chomsky N. Aspects of the theory of syntax. Cambridge, MA: MIT Press. 1965

24 Rapin I, Allen D. Developmental language disorders: nosologic considerations. In: Kirk U, ed. Neuropsychology of language, reading and spelling. New York: Academic Press. 1983

25 Powell RP, Bishop DVM. Clumsiness and perceptual problems in children with specific language impairment. Dev Med Child Neurol 1992; 34: 755–765

26 Bishop DVM. Comprehension of spoken, written and signed sentences in childhood language disorders. J Child Psychol Psychiatry 1982; 23: 1–20

27 Conti-Ramsen G, Gunn M. The development of conversational disability: a case study. Br J Disord Commun 1986; 21: 339–351

28 Conti-Ramsden G, Hensey OJ, Rosenbloom L. Management of severe language disorders: a multi-disciplinary approach. CST Bull, May 1985.

29 Corbett J, Harris R, Taylor E, Trimble M. Progressive disintegrative psychosis in childhood. J Child Psychol Psychiatry 1987; 18: 211–219

30 Landau WM, Kleffner FR. Syndrome of acquired aphasia with convulsive disorder in children. Neurology 1957; 7: 523–530

31 Gordon N. Developmental disorders of speech and language. In: Yule W, Rutter M, eds. Language development and disorders. Clinics in developmental medicine nos 101/102. Oxford: Mac Keith Press with Blackwell, 1987: pp 189–205

32 Bishop DVM. Age of onset and outcome in 'acquired aphasia with convulsive disorder' (Landau–Kleffner syndrome). Dev Med Child Neurol 1985; 27: 705–712
33 Evans-Jones LG, Rosenbloom L. Disintegrative psychosis in childhood. Dev Med Child Neurol 1978; 20: 462–470
34 Kanner L. Autistic disturbances of affective contact. Nervous child. 1943; 2: 217–250
35 American Psychiatric Association. Diagnostic and statistical manual 3rd ed revised (DSM-III-R) Washington, DC: American Psychiatric Association 1987
36 Cohen DJ, Volkmar RF, Paul R. Issues in the classification of pervasive and other developmental disorders: history and current state of nosology. J Am Acad Child Psychiatry 1986; 25: 158–161
37 Asperger H. Die 'autischen Psychopathen' im Kindesalter. Arch Psychiatr Nervenkr 1944; 117: 76–136
38 Wing L. Asperger's syndrome. J Psychol Med 1981; 11: 115–129
39 Bowman EP. Asperger's syndrome and autism: the case for a connection. Br J Psychiatry 1988; 1522: 377–382
40 Bishop DVM. Autism, Asperger's syndrome and semantic-pragmatic disorder. Where are the boundaries? Br J Disord Commun 1989; 24: 107–121
41 Howlin P, Rutter M. Treatment of autistic children. Chichester: Wiley. 1987
42 Neville A, Gunn M. A team approach to assessing and working with children with specific language difficulties. Child Language Teach Ther 1987; 3: 151–169

13

Management of atopic eczema

T. J. David

To the doctor, atopic eczema is a skin disease, but to an affected child it can be a disfiguring handicap (Table 13.1). Treatment is difficult. The condition is common. The most recently published data report that in a prospective study of 7609 infants born in five German cities in 1990, 23% had developed atopic eczema in the first year of life.[1] This chapter incorporates recent advances with existing knowledge, and discusses the practical aspects of management.

TAKING A HISTORY

Rational management is impossible without taking a careful history, yet this aspect is studiously avoided in textbooks. Questions are aimed to help answer the following questions:

Does the patient have atopic eczema, or some other disorder?

The sensation of itch and the symptom of scratching are ubiquitous in atopic eczema, and are often especially noted in a medical setting when the child's

Table 13.1 Handicapping features of atopic eczema

Sleep interruption
Disfigurement
   inflamed red skin on face
   dry ichthyotic skin
   scabs (infected eczema)
   weeping skin lesions
Teasing by other children
Abnormal body image
Treatment
   ointments, creams
   use of daytime bandaging
Unpleasant smell (severe cases)
Short stature
Limited career choice for teenagers with eczema,
     e.g. not nursing, hairdressing or food handling

clothes are removed. The absence of pruritus other than in the first three months strongly suggests an alternative diagnosis. The nature and distribution of the lesions is also important, e.g. itchy small papules or blisters on the sole of the foot and in the interdigital spaces suggest scabies rather than eczema.

Published figures of the incidence of a family history of atopy in atopic eczema, which range from 38% to 83%,[2] are gross underestimates. The complete absence of any family history of atopic disease is rare. Since 30% of the population have a first-degree relative with atopic disease, the presence of such a history is itself little help, but the absence of a family history of atopic disease would alert one to the possibility of an alternative diagnosis.

Does the patient have an underlying disorder or syndrome?

It is helpful to consider whether a patient's eczematous skin lesions are features of an underlying disorder,[3] such as an immunodeficiency state (suggested by either unusual disease severity, atypical clinical features, or a history of co-existing disorders such as recurrent infection or malabsorption) or a dysmorphic syndrome (such as the Dubowitz syndrome).

What treatment is in current use, and what effect is it perceived to have?

It is helpful to enquire about current treatment. What is being used, when and how is it being used, and what effect does it have? What parents do may bear little relation to their doctor's intentions. It is common, for example, to find parents who for no apparent reason rotate emollients, using one in the morning and evening, and another on occasions in between. Some practices may be illogical and counterproductive, such as, for example, the application of a thick layer of emulsifying ointment immediately before a thin smear of hydrocortisone. It makes sense to enquire whether the parents perceive benefit or otherwise from each treatment. This information will be useful when deciding on future treatment; it is difficult to persuade parents to use a treatment which they think is unhelpful.

What treatments have been tried in the past, and what effect have they had?

There is nothing more frustrating than to spend a long time discussing treatment with the parents of a new patient, and then to hear later from the pharmacist that when the new ointment was handed over the parents said 'Oh not that again, we've tried it and it's useless'. It is common for numerous treatments to have already been tried. It is also common that parents are unable to remember the names of most treatments, particularly those tried in the past. Fortunately, parents rarely throw away partly used tubes of ointment. Avoiding a dysfunctional consultation therefore requires a simple strategy. A routine appointment card for the first visit is accompanied by a letter which asks the family to bring to the first appointment all the creams, ointments, medicines and treatments that have been used. A suitcase may be necessary.

It is helpful to go through each item, finding out how it was used and what effect it had. There may be important information in answer to the question as to why a treatment was stopped. For example, it may have exacerbated the skin lesions. This information may be the first clue to contact sensitivity to ingredients of the preparation such as clioquinol or hydrocortisone. There may also be information which identifies a common form of dysfunctional physician behaviour, that of the doctor who changes the treatment each time the patient attends for a repeat prescription for what had been a useful and appropriate therapy.

What trigger factors have been identified?

Given the unhelpfulness of allergy tests (see later), parental observations, however unreliable where food intolerance and allergy to environmental items are concerned, are the best information available. It is helpful to discover what the parents have noticed. What triggers do the parents suspect, and why? What is the nature of the suspected reaction? What steps have the parents taken to avoid the suspected trigger? How do the parents interpret their own observations? For example, parents commonly report marked fluctuations in disease severity, a fundamental feature of atopic eczema, and many wrongly believe that this implies some external cause such as an allergy.

It is common to find a clear history of adverse reaction to an item (e.g. cow's milk) which is nevertheless being incompletely avoided, and this provides the opportunity for a therapeutic trial of a period of strict avoidance with the help of a dietitian.[4,5] The history is also useful to uncover parental false beliefs. For example, it is common to find parents who report that their child is allergic to multiple items, but when asked how they know they report that this has been proved by allergy tests, even though the history is clearly inconsistent with this.

It is common to find that some sort of dietary elimination has been tried, and is possibly in progress,[6] and it is helpful to establish why the diet was tried, how carefully it was adhered to, and whether the diet was associated with any improvement or not.

Contact triggers, such as woollen clothing or enzyme-containing washing powders, are worth enquiring about, as some patients benefit from avoidance.

What makes the condition better?

The answers to this question may occasionally give some useful clues. For example, a history that eczema markedly improves shortly after admission to hospital and deteriorates quickly after discharge points to environmental antigens such as those which come from house dust mites or pet animals. It is common to obtain a history that eczema disappears during a sunny holiday in Spain, only to relapse after return home, but although interesting, this information is of little practical value as the reasons for improvement on sunny holidays have not been identified.[7]

How does the condition affect the patient and the family?

This is a helpful area to explore. 'What is the worst feature of eczema from your point of view?' is a useful question. For example, for many families the biggest problem is sleep disturbance, and for such families the most useful therapeutic manoeuvre may be the use of a sedating H_1 histamine antagonist at bedtime. Answers to the above question can also give an indication of how well the family are coping, and may help to detect a mismatch between the severity of the disease and the parental distress.

What are the special fears and anxieties of the parents and referring doctor?

These need to be uncovered and addressed. For example, many parents fear the use of topical steroids, and this fear may result in the underuse of a safe and helpful treatment.[8] The nature of anxiety about steroids is worth exploring, so that their possible hazards can be seen in perspective. Misinformation about steroids is common amongst doctors and parents. A good example was a 4-month-old infant with facial eczema who was prescribed the potent steroid Propaderm (beclomethasone dipropionate 0.025%) with little improvement. His mother returned to the general practitioner, who this time prescribed a very mildly potent steroid, 0.5% hydrocortisone. The mother refused to take the prescription to the pharmacist; she knew hydrocortisone was far too strong for a baby's face!

In explaining the confusing and somewhat illogical subject of steroid potencies (parents are not alone in being puzzled by the reverse order of numbering, IV for the weakest and I for the most potent), it is helpful to use an analogy such as that of alcoholic beverages. Category IV steroids are mildly potent (like shandy*), category III steroids are moderately potent (like sherry), category II steroids are potent (like whisky), and category I steroids are very potent (like pure alcohol).

Even dermatologists can be confused by steroid potencies. One recent textbook[9] categorized Eumovate (clobetasone butyrate 0.05%) along with hydrocortisone as mildly potent, when it is in fact classified in the *British National Formulary*[10] as category III (moderately potent).

A common parental fear, which is usually not volunteered, is of the marked lymphadenopathy which so often accompanies atopic eczema. Most parents

---

*Mixture of equal parts of beer and lemonade.

know that big glands can be a feature of malignancy, and are reassured to learn the benign nature of dermatopathic lymphadenopathy.

What are the parents and referring doctor hoping to achieve by the consultation?

The hopes of the parents are likely to form the basis for the discussion once the child has been examined, so this is an important area to be explored. Some parents are seeking a cure. Others come with a special treatment in mind (e.g. a diet). Failure to enquire about parental wishes, hopes and fears may result in key items (to the parents) being omitted from discussion.

Other aspects

A perinatal and infant feeding history is helpful, and a full immunization history (see below) is required. Information about pet ownership should be sought.

DIAGNOSIS

Definition

It is remarkably difficult to define what does and what does not comprise atopic eczema. Textbooks of dermatology and paediatrics carefully avoid this difficult area. The largest textbook on atopic eczema,[11] which contains 50 chapters, has no section on diagnosis, and the word is not even listed in the index. Other books offer bland statements such as 'The diagnosis of typical cases of atopic dermatitis is seldom difficult'.[12] There have been a number of worthy attempts to produce diagnostic criteria,[13,14] but all are totally impractical and unsuitable for routine clinical use.

Examination of the patient

Full inspection of the skin is important even if the history only relates to one area. It is helpful to try to document the areas which are affected by eczematous lesions. Physical signs which are commonly found are a linear infraorbital fold, also called a Dennie–Morgan crease, hyperlinearity of the palms, and marked dryness and scaling of the skin. Physical signs of bacterial and viral skin infection are discussed later.

Estimation of disease severity

Objective tools for the measurement of disease severity are badly needed. At present we rely on estimates of the surface area of skin which is affected.

Unfortunately the extent of eczema (i.e. the surface area affected) gives no indication of the severity of individual skin lesions, and the estimation of severity is beset with difficulty. Should one be measuring erythema (which rapidly fluctuates), dryness, thickness, crusting or a mixture of all of these? One objective measure which looked promising from studies in adults with pruritus was the use of scratch meters,[15] but when tried in children with atopic eczema it was found that the meters were used by the patients as scratching implements, which resulted in greatly enhanced skin damage, and the meters had to be abandoned.[16]

Serological markers would be helpful. Studies of serum levels of soluble interleukin 2 receptor suggest a statistically significant correlation with disease severity[17,18] but further studies are required and at present this estimation is not easily available. In another study, a significant correlation was found between the serum concentrations of albumin or orosomucoid and measures of extent and severity,[19] but it was clear that this relationship only held for the more severe cases, and changes in these serum concentrations were not seen in mild cases.

Better definition and measurement of atopic eczema are needed, both for clinical practice and research.

MANAGEMENT

Emollients

Dryness of the skin is a prominent feature in many children with atopic eczema, and the importance of emollients is commonly stressed. However, it is far from clear exactly what is the role of emollients, and their use is poorly supported by objective studies. Furthermore, there are no comparative studies of different products, whose retail prices range from £0.80 to £30 for a 500 g tub. Given the parental effort in the application of emollients, their cost, and their detrimental effects (e.g. causing rubber to perish, or blocking drains), this is an area that warrants objective study. There is, at present, no basis for dogmatic recommendations. Some parents find emollients helpful, and others do not. The doctor's role is to help families to try different preparations such as emulsifying ointment, white soft paraffin, aqueous cream or buffered cream.

Fluctuation from day to day is a prominent feature of atopic eczema. If one is to avoid any change in eczema being wrongly attributed to benefit or harm from a new therapy, then any new topical preparation is best applied only to one area of skin, and compared with an untreated area and an area treated with a previous remedy.

Bath oils and baths

An objective basis for the use of baths oils is lacking. Their only proven effect is to make the bath slippery. Parents should be encouraged to experiment.

Although some children with eczema appear to benefit from daily or twice daily baths with the addition of a bath oil, others are helped by a reduction in the frequency of baths. Conventional advice may be hazardous. It is often suggested, for example, that emulsifying ointment should be dissolved in boiling water and then poured into the bath water, with the risk of scalds. Another suggestion is to dissolve emulsifying ointment in the bath water with an electric whisk, but this carries the risk of electrocution. In practice it is simpler, and certainly safer, to apply emulsifying ointment direct to the child's skin immediately prior to a bath.

Soap

Given the detrimental effect of soap on the stratum corneum and intercellular lipid concentration in atopic eczema,[20] there is a clear basis for considering the avoidance of soap in children with atopic eczema.

Bandages

Cotton tubular bandage can be made into mittens, and secured at the wrist using tape[21] such as Micropore tape. It is believed that such bandage can reduce damage done by scratching at night in small infants, although this has not been proven by controlled studies. A common error is to leave such bandages on during the day, which if used for prolonged periods can interfere with an infant's motor development. Prolonged use of bandaging day and night should be avoided because it can result in flexion contractures of the digits.

Medicated bandages

Medicated bandages contain zinc paste, with or without calamine, clioquinol, coal tar paste or ichthammol. It is uncommon to find parents who are willing to persist with this messy and limited approach, and it is hard to find any objective basis for their use.

Splints

Splints are cruel and should not be used.

H₁ receptor antagonists

There is evidence from studies performed in sleep laboratories that sedatives, both with and without H_1 receptor antagonist activity, reduce the first (nodding-off) phase of sleep, and may therefore be most useful in helping an eczematous child to fall asleep. If compared with adults, children are relatively resistant to the sedative effects of H_1 receptor antagonists, and startlingly large doses are required (e.g for trimeprazine tartrate, up to 30 mg per night in children up to 12 months of age, and up to 50 mg per night in those over 12 months). The most sedating H_1 receptor antagonists are trimeprazine, promethazine and chlorpheniramine; indeed trimeprazine is commonly used in paediatric surgery for premedication. All three agents are best given an hour or more before bedtime. All suffer from the practical drawback that they produce drowsiness the next morning, which may exclude their use in children of school age. Since loss of sleep is often identified by parents of eczematous children as their single biggest problem, the regular use of bedtime sedatives is often invaluable.

There is no evidence that the older sedating H_1 receptor antagonists (e.g. trimeprazine) have any anti-pruritic action in atopic eczema. Their sole action in atopic eczema is to cause sedation. Daytime use should be avoided. It simply serves to decrease concentration and increase the level of irritability. The newer non-sedating H_1 receptor antagonists are not likely to be helpful.

Bacterial skin infection

Despite textbook statements to the contrary, secondary bacterial infection is common in children with atopic eczema. In a prospective study of 190 children with atopic eczema, 40% had exacerbations of their eczema due to bacterial infection in a one-year period.[22] The physical signs suggestive of bacterial infection are pustules, crusting, or a weeping discharge. When atopic eczema suddenly worsens, bacterial infection should always be suspected. In most cases of infection one can recover *Staphylococcus aureus* from skin swabs, with the addition of the Lancefield group A β-haemolytic *Streptococcus* in about 50% of cases.

Since all subjects with atopic eczema are colonized with *Staphylococcus aureus* on the skin, the recovery of this organism from a skin swab cannot be taken as evidence of infection. Obtaining specimens for bacteriology is useful, however, to detect methicillin-resistant staphylococci.

Treatment with an oral (rather than a topical) antistaphylococcal antibiotic is essential. In Manchester, over 20% of staphylococcal isolates are resistant to erythromycin, which leaves flucloxacillin or a cephalosporin (e.g. cefadroxil) as the antibiotics of choice.

Recurrent bacterial infection

Recurrence of infection is a major practical problem, and in one prospective study recurrence of infection occurred within three months of a previous episode of infection in 30% of cases.[22] There are no proven methods for the prevention of such recurrences, and it therefore makes sense to try to obtain as much control as possible of the eczema, in the hope that this will reduce the chances of a further episode of infection. Approaches which have been used in the past to prevent recurrent infections have included antiseptics (such as triclosan 2%) in the bath water (unproven benefit), washing clothing and bedding (unproven benefit), intranasal chlorhexidine hydrochloride 0.1% and neomycin sulphate 0.5% cream (unproven benefit), topical steroid–antiseptic or steroid–antibiotic combinations (unproven benefit), and long-term anti-staphylococcal antibiotics (risk of acquisition of methicillin-resistant strains of *Staphylococcus aureus*). Where a child has recurrent infections with the Lancefield group A β-haemolytic *Streptococcus*, there may be a case for prolonged (e.g. 6 months) treatment with oral phenoxymethylpenicillin.

Paronychia

Paronychia is common, and it usually settles spontaneously, with or without drainage of pus. Occasionally required are dry dressings, oral antibiotics (if there is fever or evidence of systemic infection), and on rare occasions surgical drainage may be needed. An undocumented observation is that the incidence of paronychia is increased where the parents are obsessional about keeping the child's fingernails short.

Herpes simplex virus (HSV) skin infection

Initial (primary) infections

Textbooks assert that children with atopic eczema have increased susceptibility to infection with HSV, but there is no evidence for this. Indeed, in a controlled study, it was found that 23 out of 113 children (20%) with atopic eczema had neutralizing antibodies to HSV, compared with 34 of 113 matched controls (30%), an insignificant difference.[23] Children with atopic eczema are no more likely than normal children to become infected with the virus. However, whereas the initial infection with HSV in normal children usually consits of a self-limiting gingivostomatitis, in children with atopic eczema the initial infection may be in the skin, causing eczema herpeticum.[24] On rare occasions this can result in death, and this is usually attributable to secondary bacterial infection, a failure to make the correct diagnosis, or an undetected underlying immune deficiency state such as the Wiskott–Aldrich syndrome or IgG_2 deficiency.[25]

The key physical sign of HSV skin infection is the presence of vesicles. In an initial infection these are scattered, thin-walled lesions containing clear fluid at first. After a day or two, however, the fluid becomes turbid due to the presence of white cells, and the lesions then look pustular. These pustules often have a characteristic central depression and are described as umbilicated.

Recurrences of HSV skin infection

After recovery from an initial infection with HSV, recurrent infections are common but have a different appearance and are not accompanied by severe systemic illness. In recurrences the vesicles are confluent and quickly rupture, leaving a patch of inflamed skin that may be difficult to distinguish from ordinary eczematous lesions. These recurrences are particularly common on the face, but they can occur anywhere on the body and the site of the recurrence may vary in an individual patient.

Treatment of HSV skin infection in children with eczema

Treatment of eczema herpeticum is aimed mainly at preventing secondary bacterial infection. For recurrences of HSV and less severe episodes of initial infections, this is all that is required. Where there are signs suggestive of secondary bacterial infection, an oral antistaphylococcal antibiotic is indicated. In severe cases of initial infection, when there is a fever and general malaise, admission to a hospital and intravenous treatment with the antiviral agent acyclovir (5 mg/kg every 8 hours for 3–5 days) may be required. Some are liberal with the use of oral acyclovir (100 mg × 5 daily under 2 years; 200 mg × 5 daily over 2 years) for all initial infections, but this is not required for less severe cases, and it is unsuitable for severe cases because of unreliable absorption of the drug from the gastrointestinal tract.

Topical steroids

Topical steroid therapy is dogged by uncertainty. It is impossible to predict how much steroid will be absorbed in an individual case, although it is established that steroid absorption is enhanced in the very young, in the presence of eczema, and in certain skin sites. Thus it is impossible to state how much topical steroid can be applied before there is a risk of adverse effects from systemic absorption. The major concern with systemic absorption is growth stunting. The finding that of children with atopic eczema which is sufficiently severe to warrant regular hospital follow-up, 20% have short stature,[26] the cause of which is uncertain, leaves no room for complacency about the use of topical steroids. An unfortunate paradox is that it is the child with the most severe and extensive disease who needs steroid therapy most and is by the same token most likely to experience side effects. To withhold topical steroids in such patients for fear of side effects from systemic absorption is unreasonable. Indeed, in a very small number of patients who are unresponsive to all conventional treatment, life is tolerable only with the aid of regular systemic steroids.

In view of serious uncertainty about the safety of topical steroids, it is remarkable that not all adhere to a basic principle of treatment, namely to use the least potent preparation as sparingly as possible.[10] The first choice is 1% hydrocortisone ointment; more potent preparations are not needed for most children with atopic eczema. When other steroid preparations are used then it is advisable to check the potency, in order to avoid confusion caused by the different potencies of topical steroids, and the effect on skin absorption (and consequently potency) of substances present in the vehicle (e.g. 10% urea). Most parents think that topical steroids are dangerous, and thus any prescription must be accompanied by an explanation of the different potencies. The dryness of the skin in most cases of atopic eczema means that it is preferable to use steroid ointments rather than creams.

Potent topical steroids

An alternative and quite widely used but potentially hazardous strategy is to start treatment with a potent steroid, and after a few days change to a weaker preparation. This has the advantage of a quick response to treatment, but carries the serious risk that the parents will over-use the potent steroid, leading to skin atrophy or striae. In practice the strategy seems to be more honoured in the breach than the observance, parents either being too frightened to use the potent steroid at all or using it liberally, oblivious to the hazards. Implicit in this approach is the need to issue an unambiguous warning to the parents and the general practitioner regarding the hazards of prolonged use of potent or very potent topical steroids.

In older children it is common to see severe and heavily lichenified patches of eczema confined to the front of the knees, the wrists, and the ankles. Such lesions may not respond well to mildly potent steroids, and in this situation it makes no sense to withhold a moderately potent preparation because of fear of skin atrophy.

Total steroid load

One must remember that topical steroids applied to the skin may only be part of the total load of steroids received by the child. Those who have co-existing asthma or rhinitis may well be receiving additional topical steroids.

Antiseptic–steroid combinations

Combinations of the antiseptic clioquinol and a steroid are widely used, but there is no proof that such combinations are more effective than the steroid alone. Apart from the extra expense, clioquinol causes a permanent yellow–brown staining of clothing, and there is a theoretical hazard from percutaneous absorption.

IMMUNIZATION

Atopic eczema is often wrongly used as an excuse to withhold vaccination, particularly MMR vaccination (because of its measles component) and pertussis vaccination. Details of vaccination should be obtained when a full history is taken at the first visit, and any misinformation corrected and missing immunization provided.

BCG immunization poses a special problem, because although there is no published data, it is clear that BCG can cause very severe and prolonged (2 to 3 months or more) flare-ups of pre-existing atopic eczema. It is not known whether there are any special risks of neonatal BCG immunization in a child from an atopic family.

AVOIDABLE TRIGGER FACTORS

It may be worth trying to avoid factors which trigger or exacerbate atopic eczema, but identification of these factors is often difficult. Unfortunately, laboratory investigations such as eosinophil count, serum IgE level, and radioallergosorbent tests (RAST), are not helpful, nor are skin prick tests.[27] The lack of any valid tests for food allergy[5] has led to the development of a number of allergy clinics that use unproven methods of diagnosis and treatment such as radionics, pulse testing, urine therapy, lymphocyte cytotoxicity testing, end point titration, intradermal testing, and sublingual neutralization therapy.[28]

Fabric conditioners and washing powders

It is sometimes reported that eczema is exacerbated by the use of fabric conditioners or enzyme-containing washing powders in certain children with atopic eczema.

Clothing

It is often reported by parents that skin contact with woollen clothing can exacerbate atopic eczema in childhood. The advice that pure cotton clothing must be used is often given, but for most children polyester–cotton mixtures appear to be tolerated without difficulty.

Heat

Heat is a prominent trigger factor in most children with atopic eczema, and many parents find it helpful to keep the bedroom and sometimes the whole house at a cool temperature. Interestingly, there is a small minority of children with atopic eczema who crave warmth, and I have seen two cases of erythema ab igne in children with atopic eczema who habitually leant against hot radiators.

Environmental antigens: dust mites, grass and grass pollen, and pets

There is a singular dearth of objective data on the importance of these antigens in childhood atopic eczema, although there is no lack of anecdotes suggesting that these items, acting alone or together, may be an important contributory factor in some cases.

Current management is at best pure guesswork. Most children with atopic eczema over the age of two years possess IgE antibodies to all the above antigens, so that tests to detect these IgE antibodies (in the skin: skin prick tests, in the circulation: RAST tests) are in practice unhelpful. It is a regrettable fact that we have no test which can identify which patients will benefit from avoidance regimens.[27] This is especially unfortunate if one considers the invasiveness of removing pets (and the careful cleaning of carpets, furniture and clothing which must accompany the dispatch of the pet if the antigen is to be avoided), and the expense of rigorous house dust mite avoidance measures, where drastic steps such as removal of the bedroom carpet, bedroom toys and clothing, and replacement of divan beds (which cannot be sealed) appear to be pre-requisites for there to be any real chance of benefit. The lack of controlled trials of the clinical efficacy of various measures designed to reduce exposure to environmental antigens is a major handicap.

Intolerance to food and food additives

Study of this area is handicapped by the lack of useful simple objective tests to indicate whether a subject is or is not intolerant to foods or food additives, or to indicate which food or food additive is worth avoiding.[5] Given the multiplicity of possible mechanisms, not all of which are immunological, it seems inconceivable that any such test will ever appear. At present the best test is the double-blind placebo-controlled challenge, but unfortunately this suffers from a large number of major drawbacks, both theoretical and practical, which are discussed in detail elsewhere.[5] A common error, and an unfortunate and prominent feature of many studies, is to equate a positive blind challenge with benefit from an elimination diet. Just because a child experiences erythema an hour after ingestion of, for example, banana, is no guarantee that the child's eczema will benefit if bananas are strictly avoided.

At present we have no evidence from controlled studies of any long-term benefit from dietary avoidance regimens in atopic eczema. Indeed, such evidence as we have, suggests that there is no long-term benefit. In one follow-up study, the outcome one year after a trial of a particularly rigorous dietary regimen showed that those in whom a diet was associated with initial improvement, those in whom a diet was not associated with benefit, and those whose parents were unable to cope with a diet were all markedly improved.[29] The outcome was equally good in all three groups. There was some suggestion of short term benefit from simple egg and milk avoidance[30] although a subsequent study failed to confirm this.[31] There is also some uncontrolled data to show benefit associated with a few foods[29,32] or a so-called elemental diet,[16] but it is impossible to tell how much of this benefit was due to a placebo effect. This is a serious handicap, given the well-established placebo effect of diets in the treatment of a variety of childhood disorders.

The role of the dietitian

The dietitian has three roles in this context. One is to ensure that the resulting diet is nutritionally adequate,[33] and prevent potential deficiency states by recommending appropriate amounts of infant milk formula, and supplements of calcium, vitamins and so on. Another role is to advise the parents how to avoid specific food ingredients, particularly in manufactured foods, and if appropriate to provide recipes to help in the preparation and inclusion of unusual or unfamiliar ingredients. The third role of the dietitian is to give suggestions as to how to make the diet practical and palatable, and to suggest recipes for the use of a limited range of foods (e.g. how to make biscuits with potato flour).

Calcium

Cow's milk is an important source of calcium, and avoidance of cow's milk and its products carries a risk of an inadequate intake of calcium.[34]

Protein, energy

Milk, eggs, fish, meat, wheat, and their respective manufactured food products, are important sources of protein and energy. Avoidance of these without the provision of alternative sources of protein and energy runs the risk of an inadequate intake; growth failure and serious malnutrition are well-documented sequelae of unsupervised and inappropriate dietary elimination.[35,36]

Iodine

Cow's milk and dairy products are an important source of dietary iodine. A child has been reported in whom the unsupervised exclusion of cow's milk products and a number of other items from the diet, coupled with the consumption of large amounts of soya milk (which has itself been reported to cause hypothyroidism by increasing faecal loss of thyroxine), resulted in hypothyroidism and growth failure due to dietary iodine deficiency.[37]

Situations in which elimination diets may be especially risky

Elimination diets may pose special nutritional problems. Situations where there is a special risk are listed in Table 13.2. Unfortunately not all hospital or community clinics have easy access to a dietitian, and many dietitians are unfamiliar with the dietary management of atopic eczema.

Table 13.2   Situations in which elimination diets may be especially risky

---

Unsupervised diets — risk of malnutrition

Parental obsession — risk of inappropriate escalation of dietary avoidance

Chronic disease prior to diagnosis, or concurrent chronic disease such as severe atopic eczema. Child's nutrient requirements may be increased

Malabsorption or enteropathy — risk of malabsorption of nutrients

Child avoiding sunlight — risk of vitamin D deficiency compounding the effects of a low calcium intake.

Where a child is already on a diet which excludes multiple foods, e.g. vegan or macrobiotic diet

---

MEASUREMENTS AND INVESTIGATIONS

Height and weight

The association between short stature and atopic eczema[26] means that it makes sense to measure the height and weight of children with atopic eczema who regularly attend a clinic.

Skin swabs for bacteriology

The skin of *all* children with atopic eczema is colonized with *Staphylococcus aureus*, so the discovery of this organism in a skin swab is of no diagnostic value. In a child with suspected bacterial infection (see above), a swab for bacteriology is performed to detect antibiotic resistant strains of *Staphylococcus aureus*, and to detect the Lancefield group A β-haemolytic *Streptococcus*.

Skin swabs for herpes simplex virus (HSV)

Where HSV is present in the skin, it can be grown quickly and easily in tissue culture, and results are usually positive within 24 hours. If flare-ups of atopic eczema can be identified to result from recurrent HSV skin infection, then the patient can be spared from irrelevant therapy (e.g. diets). In theory the typical clusters of vesicles should be easily identified. In practice these easily rupture, and the resulting inflamed patch of skin may not be easily differentiated from an uncomplicated patch of atopic eczema.

Immunodeficiency

The association between atopic eczema and immunodeficiency means that the latter should be sought in the presence of certain features such as unusual disease severity, abnormal or unusual infections, failure to thrive, and

malabsorption. The appropriate immunological investigatiọngs (e.g. measurement of IgG, IgA, IgM, IgG subclasses, IgE, complement, T and B cell, and
phagocyte function) and haematological investigations (e.g. neutrophil count,
platelet count, platelet volume) should be discussed with the local laboratory.

Serum IgE concentration

It is difficult to find an indication for performing this test in a child with
atopic eczema. Almost all cases have elevated serum IgE concentrations.
Previous reports to the contrary are the result of inadequate age-related
normal data, and even on occasions the use of adult normal ranges.
Exceptions to this rule are few; some of these cases have an immunodeficiency.

In infancy, there can occasionally be difficulty in distinguishing between
the atopic and non-atopic fractions of seborrhoeic dermatitis, and in theory
measurement of the serum IgE concentration might help to identify the
atopic fraction.[38,39] In practice, the natural history of the disease enables
identification of the atopic fraction without recourse to any investigations.

Tests for specific IgE antibodies

These can be sought in the skin by skin prick testing or in the circulation by
radioimmunological methods (e.g. RAST testing). The problems of these tests
are discussed in detail elsewhere,[5,27] but in short these tests are beset with
problems which include lack of standardization, and a high incidence of false
positive and false negative results. The greatest problem is that there are as yet
no objective data to suggest that the use of these tests can predict the outcome
of antigen avoidance measures. It is hard to justify the continued use of these
tests in routine clinical practice.

Measurement of the serum albumin concentration

This is indicated in exceptionally severe cases, in whom hypoproteinaemia
and oedema can occasionally be a feature.

EXCEPTIONALLY SEVERE CASES

Even with the most careful application of conventional treatment of atopic
eczema in childhood, there remain a number of children with intractable
and handicapping eczema. The management of these cases is dealt with
elsewhere.[40]

PARENT AND PATIENT SUPPORT GROUPS

Parents can receive much support from contact with other parents and from
local self-help groups. In the United Kingdom, useful information for patients

and parents is obtainable from the National Eczema Society, 4 Tavistock Place, London WC1H 9RA.

KEY POINTS FOR CLINICAL PRACTICE

- Include in the history details of the current and previous treatment and its perceived effect.
- Enquire about suspected trigger factors, including information about why a factor is suspected to provoke eczema.
- To avoid confusion from spontaneous fluctuation in disease severity, new topical treatments are often best applied to only one area of skin, and compared with an untreated area and an area treated with a previous remedy.
- Loss of sleep is often identified by parents of eczematous children as their single biggest problem, and the regular use of bedtime sedatives (e.g. trimeprazine tartrate) is often invaluable.
- The physical signs suggestive of bacterial infection are pustules, crusting, or a weeping discharge. When atopic eczema suddenly worsens, bacterial infection should always be suspected, and oral antistaphylococcal antibiotics given.
- Since all subjects with atopic eczema are colonized with *Staphylococcus aureus* on the skin, the recovery of this organism from a skin swab cannot be taken as evidence of bacterial infection.
- Use the least potent topical steroid preparation as sparingly as possible. The first choice is 1% hydrocortisone ointment; more potent preparations are not needed for most children with atopic eczema.
- Elimination diets should be supervised by a dietitian, to avoid nutritional deficiency and to ensure complete avoidance of specific food items.

REFERENCES

1 Bergmann RL, Lau-Schadendorf S, Wahn U. The atopic career in childhood — the German multicenter atopy study (MAS-90). Allergy Clin Immunol News 1993; 5: 4951
2 Schultz Larsen F. Genetic aspects of atopic eczema. In: Ruzicka T, Ring J, Przybilla B, eds. Handbook of atopic eczema. Berlin: Springer, 1991: pp 15–30
3 Fritsch P, Hintner H. Immunodeficiency syndromes and atopic eczema. In Ruzicka T, Ring J, Przybilla B, eds. Handbook of atopic eczemaa. Berlin: Springer, 1991: pp 107–116
4 David TJ. Dietary treatment of atopic eczema. Arch Dis Child 1989; 64: 1506–1509
5 David TJ. Intolerance to food and food additives in childhood. Oxford: Blackwell, 1993: pp 239–280, pp 439–454
6 Webber SA, Graham-Brown RAC, Hutchinson PE, Burns DA. Dietary manipulation in childhood atopic dermatitis. Br J Dermatol 1989; 121: 91–98
7 Turner MA, Devlin J, David TJ. Holidays and atopic eczema. Arch Dis Child 1991; 66: 212–215
8 David TJ. Steroid scare. Arch Dis Child 1987; 62: 876–878
9 Marks R. Practical problems in dermatology. London: Dunitz, 1984: p 166
10 British National Formulary, No 25. London: British Medical Association and the Royal Pharmaceutical Society of Great Britain, 1993: p 413
11 Ruzicka T, Ring J, Przybilla B, eds. Handbook of atopic eczema. Berlin: Springer, 1991

12 Champion RH, Parish WE. Atopic dermatitis. In: Champion RH, Burton JL, Ebling JL, Ebling FJG, eds. Rook/Wilkinson/Ebling's Textbook of dermatology, Volume 1. 5th ed. Oxford: Blackwell, 1992: pp 589–610.

13 Hanifin JM, Rajka G. Diagnostic features of atopic dermatitis. Acta Dermato-Venereol (Stockh) 1980; 92 (suppl): 44–47

14 Svensson A, Edman B, Moller H. A diagnostic tool for atopic dermatitis based on clinical criteria. Acta Derm Venereol (Stockh) 1985; 114 (suppl): 33–40

15 Summerfield JA, Welch ME. The measurement of itch with sensitive limb movement meters. Br J Dermatol 1980; 102: 275–280

16 Devlin J, David TJ, Stanton RHJ. Elemental diet for refractory atopic eczema. Arch Dis Child 1991; 66: 93–99

17 Colver GB, Symons JA, Duff GW. Soluble interleukin 2 receptor in atopic eczema. Br Med J 1989; 298: 1426–1428

18 Wuthrich B, Joller-Jemelka H, Helfenstein U, Grob PJ. Levels of soluble interleukin-2 receptors correlate with the severity of atopic dermatitis. Dermatologica 1990; 181: 92–97

19 David TJ, Wells FE, Sharpe TC, Gibbs ACC, Devlin J. Serum levels of trace metals in children with atopic eczema. Br J Dermatol 1990; 122: 485–489

20 White MI, McEwan Jenkinson D, Lloyd DH. The effect of washing on the thickness of the stratum corneum in normal and atopic individuals. Br J Dermatol 1987; 116: 525–530

21 Atherton DJ. Your child with eczema. A guide for parents. London: Heinemann, 1985: pp 72–73

22 David TJ, Cambridge GC. Bacterial infection and atopic eczema. Arch Dis Child 1986; 61: 20–23

23 David TJ, Richmond SJ, Bailey AS. Serological evidence of herpes simplex infections in atopic eczema. Arch Dis Child 1987; 62: 416–417

24 David TJ, Longson M. Herpes simplex infections in atopic eczema. Arch Dis Child 1985; 60: 338–343

25 Ewing CI, Roper HP, David TJ, Haeney MR. Death from eczema herpeticum in a child with severe eczema, mental retardation and cataracts. J Roy Soc Med 1989; 82: 169–170

26 Kristmundsdottir F, David TJ. Growth impairment in children with atopic eczema. J Roy Soc Med 1987; 80: 9–12

27 David TJ. Conventional allergy tests. Arch Dis Child 1991; 66: 281–282

28 David TJ. Unhelpful recent developments in the diagnosis and treatment of allergy and food intolerance in children. In Dobbing J, ed. Food Intolerance. London: Baillière Tindall, 1987: pp 185–214

29 Devlin J, David TJ, Stanton RHJ. Six food diet for childhood atopic dermatitis. Acta Derm Venereol (Stockh) 1991; 71: 20–24

30 Atherton DJ, Sewell M, Soothill JF, Wells RS, Chilvers CED. A double-blind controlled crossover trial of an antigen-avoidance diet in atopic eczema. Lancet 1978; 1: 401–403

31 Nelid VS, Marsden RA, Bailes JA, Bland JM. Egg and milk exclusion diets in atopic eczema. Br J Dermatol 1986; 114: 117–123

32 Pike MG, Carter CM, Boulton P, Turner MW, Soothill, JF, Atherton DJ. Few food diets in the treatment of atopic eczema. Arch Dis Child 1989; 64: 1691–1698

33 David TJ, Waddington E, Stanton RHJ. Nutritional hazards of elimination diets in children with atopic eczeman. Arch Dis Child 1984; 59: 323–325

34 Devlin J, Stanton RHJ, David TJ. Calcium intake and cows' milk free diets. Arch Dis Child 1989; 64: 1183–1184

35 Roberts IF, West RJ, Ogilvie D, Dillon MJ. Malnutrition in infants receiving cult diets a form of child abuse. Br Med J 1979; 1: 296–298

36 Tarnow-Mordi WO, Moss C, Ross K. Failure to thrive owing to inappropriate diet free of gluten and cows' milk. Br Med J 1984; 289: 1113–1114

37 Labib M, Gama R, Wright J, Marks V, Robins D. Dietary maladvice as a cause of hypothyroidism and short stature. Br Med J 1989; 298: 232–233

38 Yates VM, Kerr REI, Mackie RM. Early diagnosis of infantile seborrhoeic dermatitis and atopic dermatitis — clinical features. Br J Dermatol 1983; 108: 633–638

39 Yates VM, Kerr REI, Frier K, Cobb SJ, Mackie RM. Early diagnosis of infantile seborrhoeic dermatitis and atopic dermatitis — total and specific IgE levels. Br J Dermatol 1983; 108: 639–645

40 David TJ. New approaches to the treatment of atopic dermatitis in childhood. Pediatr Rev Commun 1991: 5: 145–157

14

Paediatric literature review — 1992

T. J. David

ALLERGY AND IMMUNOLOGY

Shield JPH, Strobel S, Levinsky RJ et al. Immunodeficiency presenting as hypergammaglobulinaemia with IgG2 subclass deficiency. Lancet 1992; 340: 448–450. *Report of 8 patients with recurrent bacterial infections, lymphadenopathy, failure to thrive and hypergammaglobulinaemia who on further investigation were found to have IgG2 deficiency. For correspondence see p 979.*

Wheeler JG, Steiner D. Evaluation of humoral responsiveness in children. Pediatr Infect Dis J 1992; 11: 304–310. *The evaluation of a post-vaccine antibody responsive can help to evaluate possible humoral immune deficiency syndromes.*

CARDIOVASCULAR

Hypertension

Deal JE, Barratt TM, Dillon MJ. Management of hypertensive emergencies. Arch Dis Child 1992; 67: 1089–1092. *The use of labetalol and sodium nitroprusside by incremental infusion resulted in improved control of accelerated hypertension. For study of blood pressure in first 10 years of life, see Br Med J 1992; 304: 23–26; for severe narrowing of the abdominal aorta as a cause of hypertension, see Arch Dis Child 1992; 67: 501–505; for skeletal traction as a cause of hypertension, see Eur J Pediatr 1992; 151: 543–545.*

Gompels C, Savage D. Home blood pressure monitoring in diabetes. Arch Dis Child 1992; 67: 636–639. *Home blood pressure monitoring is of value in the management of diabetic children.*

COMMUNITY

Black D. Children of parents in prison. Arch Dis Child 1992; 67: 967–970. *Review.*

Partin JC, Hamill SK, Fischel JE et al. Painful defecation and fecal soiling in children. Pediatrics 1992; 89: 1007–1009. *Early effective treatment of painful defecation in infancy might reduce the incidence of chronic faecal impaction and faecal soiling in school-age children.*

St James-Roberts I. Managing infants who cry persistently. Support services need to be developed while promising leads are pursued. Br Med J 1992; 304: 997–998. *Review.*

Accidents and poisoning

Bixby-Hammett DM. Pediatric equestrian injuries. Pediatrics 1992; 89: 1173–1176. *Report of 200 000 horse-related injuries, including 208 fatalities.*

Cameron D, Bishop C, Sibert JR. Farm accidents in children. Br Med J 1992; 305: 23–25. *Farms remain a dangerous environment for children. For editorial see pp 6–7, and for report of 587 cases of glass injury, see* Br Med J *1992; 304: 360.*

Duhaime AC, Alario AJ, Lewander WJ et al. Head injury in very young children: mechanism, injury type, and ophthalmologic findings in 100 hospitalized patients younger than 2 years of age. Pediatrics 1992; 90: 179–185. *In this series of 100 children under 2 years of age who were admitted because of head injury, 24% of injuries were thought to be inflicted. Retinal haemorrhages were often, but not always, associated with inflicted injuries.*

Kemp A, Sibert JR. Drowning and near drowning in children in the United Kingdom: lessons for prevention. Br Med J 1992; 304: 1143–1146. *Report of 306 submersion incidents, with 149 deaths. See also* Arch Dis Child *1992; 67: 257–261,* Pediatrics *1992; 90: 909–913, and for bucket-related drownings see* Pediatrics *1992; 89: 1068–1071.*

Litovitz T, Manoguerra A. Comparison of pediatric poisoning hazards: an analysis of 3.8 million exposure incidents. A report from the American Association of Poison Control Centers. Pediatrics 1992; 89: 999–1006. Detailed analysis of almost 4 million reported episodes. For falling admission rates see J Epidemiol Commun Health *1992; 46: 207–210, and for review of 2382 cases of button or cylindrical battery ingestion, see pp 747–757.*

Orenstein JB, Klein BL, Ochsenschlager DW. Delayed diagnosis of pediatric cervical spine injury. Pediatrics 1992; 89: 1185–1188. *Report of 9 cases.*

Bicycle accidents and bicycle helmets

Cote TR, Sacks JJ, Lambert-Huber DA et al. Bicycle helmet use among Maryland children: effect of legislation and education. Pediatrics 1992; 89: 1216–1220. *Legislation to make bicycle helmet use compulsory was associated with an increase in helmet use from 4% to 47%. See also* Pediatrics *1992; 89: 1248–1250 and 90: 354–358*

Simpson AHRW, Mineiro J. Prevention of bicycle accidents. Injury 1992; 23: 171–173. *Children under the age of 8 years should not be allowed on public roads, and older children should only be allowed on the roads after formal training. Campaigns to increase the awareness of motorists, more dedicated roads and tracks for cycle use, and protective headgear are all desirable.*

Storo W. The role of bicycle helmets in bicycle-related injury prevention. Clin Pediatr 1992; 31: 421–427. *Review. See also pp 672–677, and Am J* Dis. Child *1992; 146: 1465–1467.*

Trippe HR. Helmets for pedal cyclists. They reduce the numbers of head injuries. Br Med J 1992; 305: 843–844. *Review. For two opposing viewpoints on the value of cycle helmets, see pp 881–883.*

Child abuse

Samuels MP, McClaughlin W, Jackson RR et al. Fourteen cases of imposed upper airway obstruction. Arch Dis Child 1992; 67: 162–170. *All cases presented as recurrent severe cyanotic episodes. For correspondence see p 1519, and also see* Lancet *1992; 340: 87 and 481.*

Wiseman MR, Vizard E, Bentovim A et al. Reliability of video taped interviews with children suspected of being sexually abused. Br Med J 1992; 304: 1089–1091. *Those with more experience of dealing with sexual abuse were better at identifying high likelihood cases. For myotonic dystrophy as a possible source of confusion see* Arch Dis Child *1992; 67: 527–528.*

Enuresis

Evans JHC, Meadow SR. Desmopressin for bed wetting: length of treatment, vasopressin secretion, and response. Arch Dis Child 1992; 67: 184–188. *A 3-month course is no more effective than 1 month; most cases relapse when treatment is stopped. For a fascinating personal account see* Lancet *1992; 340: 957–958.*

Epilepsy

Bannon MJ, Wildig C, Jones PW. Teachers' perceptions of epilepsy. Arch Dis Child 1992; 67: 1467–1471. *Most teachers did not feel confident when teaching children who had epilepsy, and few considered their knowledge of the subject to be adequate.*

Handicap

Blasco PA, Allaire JH. Drooling in the developmentally disabled: management practices and recommendations. Dev Med Child Neurol 1992; 34: 849–862. *Review.*

Shaywitz SE, Escobar MD, Shaywitz BA et al. Evidence that dyslexia may represent the lower tail of a normal distribution of reading ability. N Engl J Med 1992; 326: 145–150. *Suggests that reading difficulties, including dyslexia, occur as part of a continuum that also includes normal reading ability. For editorial see pp 192–193.*

Immunization

Benjamin CM, Chew GC, Silman AJ. Joint and limb symptoms in children after immunisation with measles, mumps, and rubella vaccine. Br Med J 1992; 304: 1075–1078. *Measles, mumps and rubella vaccine is associated with an increased risk of episodes of joint and limb symptoms, especially in girls and children under 5. For provocation paralysis after immunization see* Lancet *1992; 340: 1005–1006.*

Booy R, Aitken SJM, Taylor S et al. Immunogenicity of combined diphtheria, tetanus, and pertussis vaccine given at 2, 3, and 4 months versus 3, 5 and 9 months of age. Lancet 1992; 339: 507–510. *With an accelerated immunization schedule, maternal antibodies can have an inhibitory effect on the responses to immunization against tetanus and pertussis. For editorial see pp 526–527.*

Cartwright KAV. Vaccine against *Haemophilus influenzae b* disease. Should almost eradicate the disease if uptake is high. Br Med J 1992; 305: 485–486. *Review. See also* Lancet *1992; 340: 592–594.*

Hengster P, Schnapka J, Fille M et al. Occurrence of suppurative lymphadenitis after a change of BCG vaccine. Arch Dis Child 1992; 67: 952–955. *84 of 1950 vaccinated newborn babies developed severe suppurative lymphadenitis 3–28 weeks after vaccination with a more virulent strain of BCG. The authors reviewed their vaccination policy and came to the conclusion that, except for high-risk groups, neonatal BCG vaccination is not justified in western countries. For variations in BCG policy in the UK, see* Br Med J *1992; 305: 495–498.*

McConnochie KM, Roghmann KJ. Immunization opportunities missed among urban poor children. Pediatrics 1992; 89: 1010–1026. *The major missed opportunities were acute illness visits (64%), well child or chronic illness visits (36%) and emergency department visits (18%).*

Peter G. Childhood immunizations. N Engl J Med 1992; 327: 1794–1800. *Review.*

Thakker Y, Woods S. Storage of vaccines in the community: weak link in the cold chain? Br Med J 1992; 304: 756–758. *This study showed poor adherence to the national guidelines for vaccine storage, and exposure of vaccines to a wide range of temperatures. See also* Pediatrics *1992; 89: 193–196.*

Werzberger A, Mensch B, Kuter B et al. A controlled trial of formalin-inactivated hepatitis A vaccine in healthy children. N Engl J Med 1992; 327: 453–457. *A single dose of inactivated purified hepatitis A vaccine was well-tolerated and highly protected against clinically apparent hepatitis A. For editorial see pp 488–490.*

Infant feeding

Beeken S, Waterston T. Health service support of breast feeding — are we practising what we preach? Br Med J 1992; 305: 285–287. *Of 50 first-time breast-feeding mothers, 30 said that they were separated from their babies on the first night after birth. 82/213 (42%) of nursing professionals said that breast-fed babies were frequently given water to drink. 28 (56%) of babies had received food or water other than breast milk. Although many health workers were in favour of breast-feeding, the advice given to mothers by professionals often conflicted with optimum practice guidelines.*

Lucas A, Lockton S, Davies PSW. Randomised trial of a ready-to-feed compared with powdered formula. Arch Dis Child 1992; 67: 935–939. *Despite similar nutrient composition of the two formulas, those fed the powdered formula had significantly increased body weight and skinfold thickness gains, and became significantly heavier than a further group of 20 breast-fed infants by 3 and 6 months. The data suggest that errors in reconstitution of formula from powder might be the main cause for the growth differences observed.*

Lucas A, Morley R, Cole TJ et al. Breast milk and subsequent intelligence quotient in children born preterm. Lancet 1992; 339: 261–264. *Suggests beneficial effect of human milk on neurodevelopment. For correspondence, see pp 612–614, 744–745 and 926–927.*

Martines JC, Rea M, Zoysa I. Breast feeding in the first six months. No need for extra fluids. Br Med J 1992; 304: 1068–1069. *Review. See also* Pediatrics *1992; 90: 760–766.*

Lead and its effects

Baghurst PA. McMichael AJ, Wigg NR et al. Environmental exposure to lead and children's intelligence at the age of seven years. The Port Pirie Cohort Study. New Engl J Med 1992; 327: 1279–1284. *Low-level exposure to lead during early childhood is inversely associated with neuropsychological development through the first 7 years of life. For editorial, see pp 1308–1310, and for neuroendocrine effects see* Pediatrics *1992; 90: 186–189.*

Bellinger DC, Stiles KM, Needleman HL. Low-level lead exposure, intelligence and academic achievement: a long-term follow-up study. Pediatrics 1992; 90: 855–861. *Slightly elevated blood levels around the age of 24 months are associated with intellectual and academic performance deficits from the age of 10. See editorial pp 995–997, and also* Am J Dis Child *1992; 146: 1278–1281.*

Sayre JW, Ernhart CB. Control of lead exposure in childhood. Are we doing it correctly? Am J Dis Child 1992; 146: 1275–1278. *Review. For study of lead intoxication in infancy, see* Pediatrics *1992; 89: 87–90*

Wasserman G, Graziano JH, Factor-Litvak P. Independent effects of lead exposure and iron deficiency anemia on developmental outcome at age 2 years. J Pediatr 1992; 121: 695–703. *The brain is vulnerable to the affects of both lead exposure and anaemia before 2 years of age. On a global basis, the developmental consequences of anaemia may exceed those of lead exposure.*

Sudden infant death syndrome (SIDS)

Hunt CE, Shannon DC. Sudden infant death syndrome and sleeping position. Pediatrics 1992; 90: 115–118. *Review. See also* Pediatrics *1992; 89: 1120–1126 and* Dev Med Child Neurol *1992; 34: 916–925.*

Matthews TG. The autonomic nervous system — a role in sudden infant death syndrome. Arch Dis Child 1992; 67: 654–656. *Review.*

Ponsonby A-L, Dwyer T, Gibbons LE et al. Thermal environment and sudden infant death syndrome: case-control study. Br Med J 1992; 304: 277–282. *Overheating and prone sleeping position are independently associated with an increased risk of the sudden infant death syndrome. For editorial, see pp 265–266, and see also* Arch Dis Child *1992; 67: 171–177. For climatic temperature and regional variation of SIDS in Australia see* Med J Aust *1992; 156: 246–251.*

Wigfield RE, Fleming, PJ, Berry PJ et al. Can the fall in Avon's sudden infant death rate be explained by changes in sleeping position? Br Med J 1992; 304: 282–283. *The fall in mortality can be almost entirely accounted for by the reduction in prone sleeping.*

Surveillance/screening

Glascoe FP, Byrne KE, Ashford LG et al. Accuracy of the Denver-II development screening. Pediatrics 1992; 89: 1211–1225. *Almost half the children without developmental problems received suspect scores on this scale, although the test identified correctly 83% of children with developmental problems and learning disabilities. For editorial, see pp 1253–1255, and for an overview of the restandardized test see pp 91–97.*

McClelland RJ, Watson DR, Lawless V et al. Reliability and effectiveness of screening for hearing loss in high risk neonates. Br Med J 1992; 304: 806–809. *Routine screening for hearing loss by brainstem auditory evoked potential testing in high-risk neonates is reliable and cost-effective, and routine testing of these infants would result in over half of all children with severe bilateral perinatal sensorineural hearing impairment being identified by 2 months of age. For use of auditory response cradle see* Arch Dis Child *1992; 67: 911–919.*

Voss LD, Mulligan J, Betts PR, Wilkin TJ. Poor growth in school entrants as an index of organic disease: the Wessex growth study. Br Med J 1992; 305: 1400–1402. *180 of 14 346 children at school entry had a height below the third centile. 25 were already known to have a chronic organic disease; investigations revealed a further 7 conditions which had been missed at the school entry medical examination.*

DERMATOLOGY

Darmstadt GL, Schmidt P, Wechsler DS et al. Dermatitis as a presenting sign of cystic fibrosis. Arch Dermatol 1992; 128: 1358–1364. *A reminder that cystic fibrosis can present with a florid red scaly rash, combined with severe failure to thrive, hypoproteinaemia and oedema. For editorial see pp 1389–1390.*

McDonagh AJG, Wright AI, Cork MJ et al. Nickel sensitivity: the influence of ear piercing and atopy. Br J Dermatol 1992; 126: 16–18. *Ear piercing seems to induce nickel allergy which may result in lifelong morbidity and difficulty in employment. For nickel allergy from bed-wetting alarm resulting in misdiagnosis of child abuse, see* Pediatrics *1992; 90: 458–460.*

ENDOCRINOLOGY

Counts DR, Cutler GB. Pathogenesis and therapy of precocious puberty. Curr Opin Pediatr 1992; 4: 674–678. *Review.*

Ritzen EM. Adrenogenital syndrome. Curr Opin Pediatr 1992; 4: 661–667. *Review.*

Shah A, Stanhope R, Matthew D. Hazards of pharmacological tests of growth hormone secretion in childhood. Br Med J 1992; 304: 173–174. *Overtreatment of hypoglycaemia after insulin or glugacon tests of growth hormone secretion may result in cerebral oedema.*

Spitz L, Bhargave RK, Grant DB et al. Surgical treatment of hyperinsulinaemic hypoglycaemia in infancy and childhood. Arch Dis Child 1992; 67: 201–205. *Report of 21 cases.*

Zwaan CM, Odink RJH, Delemarre-Van de Waal HA et al. Acute adrenal insufficiency after discontinuation of inhaled corticosteroid therapy. Lancet 1992; 340: 1289–1290. *Hypothalamic-pituitary-adrenal axis suppression is a serious complication in children treated for asthma with normal-dose long-term inhaled steroids.*

Diabetes

Hammond P, Wallis S. Cerebral oedema in diabetic ketoacidosis. Still puzzling — and often fatal. Br Med J 1992; 305: 203–204. *Editorial.*

Kalter-Leibovici O, Laron Z. Vascular complications of childhood diabetes mellitus. Curr Opin Pediatr 1992; 4: 685–694. *Review.*

MacFarlane A. Diabetes in puberty. Arch Dis Child 1992; 67: 569–573. *Review.*

Robertson RP. Pancreatic and islet transplantation for diabetes — cures or curiosities? N Engl J Med 1992; 327: 1861–1868. *Review.*

Growth

Brook CGD. Who's for growth hormone? Growth hormone should be given only to short children with demonstrably inadequate secretion of the natural hormone. Br Med J 1992; 304: 131–132. *Review.*

Joss EE, Temperli R, Mullis PE. Adult height in constitutionally tall stature: accuracy of five different height prediction methods. Arch Dis Child 1992; 67: 1357–1362. *No method is best, and the predictions have large confidence limits.*

Kida K, Ito T, Hayashi M et al. Urinary excretion of human growth hormone in children with short stature: correlation with pituitary secretion of human growth hormone. J Pediatr 1992; 120: 233–237. *Measurement of growth hormone in the urine can be used to screen for its deficiency.*

Obesity

Garrow JS. Treatment of obesity. Lancet 1992; 340: 409–413. *Review. For review of pathogenesis, see pp 403–408, and for long-term effects for adolescent obesity, see Engl J Med 1992; 327: 1350–1355 and 1379–1380.*

ENT

Berman S, Nuss R, Boark R et al. Effectiveness of continuous vs. intermittent amoxycillin to prevent episodes of otitis media. Pediatr Infect Dis J 1992; 11: 63–67. *Children with 3 or more episodes of otitis media in the preceding 6 months were randomly assigned to receiving amoxycillin either twice a day every day for the 4 months or twice a day only when they developed nasal congestion, runny nose or cough. Continuous amoxycillin was more effective than intermittent treatment in preventing otitis media episodes in patients 12 months or older.*

Fortnum HM. Hearing impairment after bacterial meningitis: a review. Arch Dis Child 1992; 67: 1128–1133. *Review. See also pp 1111–1112.*

Gibbin KP. Paediatric cochlear implantation. Arch Dis Child 1992; 67: 669–674. *Review.*

Putnam PE, Orenstein SR. Hoarseness in a child with gastroesophageal reflux. Acta Paediatr 1992; 81: 635–636. *Report of a case in which treatment of well-documented gastro-oesophageal reflux and oesophagitis in a young girl with hoarseness and nocturnal cough led to resolution of these symptoms.*

Wald ER. Sinusitis in children. N Engl J Med 1992; 326: 319–323. *Review.*

Glue ear

Anonymous. The treatment of persistent glue ear in children. Are surgical interventions effective in combating disability from glue ear? Effective Health Care 1992; 4: 1–15. Published by School of Public Health, University of Leeds, Leeds LS2 9LN. *Critical review, which questions whether there is a causal link between glue ear and significant disability, questions the current high rate of surgical intervention in the UK, and advocates a period of 'watchful waiting' prior to surgery to ensure that surgery is only performed where it is really needed. See also Lancet 1992; 340: 1324–1325.*

Maw AR. Using tympanometry to detect glue ear in general practice. Overreliance will lead to overtreatment. Br Med J 1992; 304: 67–68. *Review. For review of swimming and grommets see Br Med J 1992; 304: 198.*

GASTROENTEROLOGY

Booth IW. Silent gastro-oesophageal reflux: how much do we miss? Arch Dis Child 1992; 67: 1325–1327. *Reviews. For suggestion that thickening of feeds causes increased coughing in infants with reflux, see J Pediatr 1992; 121: 913–915.*

Fakhoury K, Durie PR, Levison H et al. Meconium ileus in the absence of cystic fibrosis. Arch Dis Child 1992; 67: 1204–1206. *8 of 37 newborn infants with meconium ileus did not have cystic fibrosis — a reminder that the former is not always associated with the latter.*

Hakeem V, Fifield R, Al-Bayaty HF et al. Salivary IgA antigliadin antibody as a marker for coeliac disease. Arch Dis Child 1992; 67: 724–727. *Suggests that this may provide a rapid, non-invasive method of screening.*

Judd RH. *Helicobacter pylori*, gastritis, and ulcers in pediatrics. Adv Pediatr 1992; 39: 283–306. *Review. See also Arch Dis Child 1992; 67: 940–943.*

Cystic fibrosis

Atlas AB, Orenstein SR, Orenstein DM. Pancreatitis in young children with cystic fibrosis. J Pediatr 1992; 120: 756–759. *Pancreatitis should be considered as a possible cause of abdominal pain in pancreatic-sufficient children with cystic fibrosis.*

Pyloric stenosis

Vanderwinden JM, Mailleux P, Schiffmann SN et al. Nitric oxide synthase activity in infantile hypertrophic pyloric stenosis. N Engl J Med 1992; 327: 511–515. *Suggests that a lack of nitric oxide synthase in pyloric tissue causes pylorospasm in pyloric stenosis. For editorial, see pp 558–560.*

GENETIC AND MALFORMATIONS

Genetics

Prockop DJ. Mutations in collagen genes as a cause of connective-tissue diseases. N Engl J Med 1992; 326: 540–546. *Review.*

Malformations

Bos AP, Broers CJM, Hazebroek FWJ et al. Avoidance of emergency surgery in newborn infants with trisomy 18. Lancet 1992; 339: 913–917. *Rapid confirmation of Edwards' syndrome by karyotyping of a bone marrow aspirate is important, because surgery may then be withheld. For editorial, see pp 902–903 and correspondence see p 1235.*

Czeizel, AE, Dudas I. Prevention of the first occurrence of neural-tube defects by periconceptional vitamin supplementation. N Engl J Med 1992; 327: 1832–1835. *Periconceptional vitamin use decreases the incidence of a first occurrence of neural tube defects. See editorial pp 1875–1877, and for hot baths as a risk factor for neural tube defects see* Dev Med Child Neurol *1992; 34: 661–675.*

Lee B, Ramirez F. Marfan syndrome. Curr Opin Pediatr 1992; 4: 965–971. *Review. For relationship with mutations of the fibrillin gene, see* N Engl J Med *1992; 326: 905–909.*

Schumacher R, Mai A, Gutjahr P. Association of rib anomalies and malignancy in childhood. Eur J Pediatr 1992; 151: 432–434. *Rib anomalies were found in 22% of children with tumours and 5% of normal children.*

Sharland M, Burch M, McKenna WM et al. A clinical study of Noonan syndrome. Arch Dis Child 1992; 67: 178–183. *Review of 151 cases. See also* Lancet *1992; 340: 22–23*

HÆMATOLOGY

Adams R, McKie V, Nichols F et al. The use of transcranial ultrasonography to predict stroke in sickle cell disease. N Engl J Med 1992; 326: 605–610. *Transcranial ultrasonography can identify the children with sickle cell disease who are at highest risk for cerebral infarction. Periodic ultrasound examinations and the selective use of transfusion therapy could make the primary prevention of stroke an achievable goal. For editorial see pp 637–638, and for report of strokes in 17 out of 310 patients see* J Pediatr *1992; 120: 360–366.*

Calvo EB, Galindo AC, Aspres NB. Iron status in exclusively breast-fed infants. Pediatrics 1992; 90: 375–379. *The results indicate that breast-fed infants require supplemental iron from the fourth month of life.*

Eden OB, Lilleyman JS. Guidelines for management of idiopathic thrombocytopenic purpura. Arch Dis Child 1992; 67: 1056–1058. *Review.*

Evans DIK. Bone marrow transplantation for thalassaemia major. J Clin Pathol 1992; 45: 553–555. *Review.*

Hann IM. Myelodysplastic syndromes. Arch Dis Child 1992; 67: 962–966. *Review.*

O'Sullivan J, Chatuverdi R, Bennett MK et al. Protein S deficiency: early presentation and pulmonary hypertension. Arch Dis Child 1992; 67: 960–961. *Any child with unexplained pulmonary hypertension and evidence of arterial thrombus should be considered as having protein S deficiency until proved otherwise.*

Rao SP, Miller ST, Cohen BJ. Transient aplastic crisis in patients with sickle cell disease. B19 parvovirus studies during a 7-year period. Am J

Dis Child 1992; 146: 1328–1330. *70% of cases of transient aplastic crisis were caused by parvovirus infection. For details of nosocomial spread of parvovirus, see* Lancet *1992; 339: 107–109 and* Communic Dis Rep *1992; 2: 237.*

Whittle MJ. Rhesus haemolytic disease. Arch Dis Child 1992; 67: 65–68. *Review.*

INFECTIOUS DISEASE

Cartwright K, Reilly S, White D et al. Early treatment with parenteral penicillin in meningococcal disease. Br Med J 1992; 305: 143–147. *Parenteral antibiotic given by general practitioners was associated with a reduction in mortality (from 9 to 5%) and the authors recommend that family doctors should give benzylpenicillin promptly, preferably intravenously, whenever meningococcal disease is suspected. For editorial see pp 133–134, for correspondence see pp 420, 523–524 and 774, and for similar study which reported that none of 13 patients given parenteral penicillin before admission died, compared with 8 deaths (24%) in 33 patients admitted without such treatment, see pp 141–143.*

Chomel BB. Zoonoses of house pets other than dogs, cats and birds. Pediatr Infect Dis J 1992; 11: 479–487. *Review.*

Epstein M, Pearson ADJ, Hudson SJ et al. Necrobacillosis with pancytopenia. Arch Dis Child 1992; 67: 958–959. *A report of 2 young children with a septicaemic illness, in which the severe suppurative multisystem illness was complicated by pancytopenia and resulted in referral to an oncology unit.*

Goren A, Freier S, Passwell JH. Lethal toxic encephalopathy due to childhood shigellosis in a developed country. Pediatrics 1992; 89: 1189–1193. *The mortality from shigellosis in a developed country is due primarily to a toxic encephalopathy, and the authors report 15 such cases.*

Guerina NG. Clinicopathological conference. N Engl J Med 1992; 326: 1480–1489. *Detailed report of a 6-year-old with encephalopathy due to cat-scratch disease.*

Joce R, Wood D, Brown D et al. Paralytic poliomyelitis in England and Wales, 1985–91. Br Med J 1992; 305: 79–82. *Of 21 cases, 13 were vaccine-associated (9 recipient and 4 contact), 5 were imported cases and in 3 the source of infection was unknown.*

La Via WV, Marks MI, Stutman HR et al. Respiratory syncytial virus puzzle: clinical features, pathophysiology, treatment, and prevention. J Pediatr 1992; 121: 503–510. *Review. For prevention of nosocomial infection, see* Lancet *1992; 340: 1071–1073 and 1079–1083.*

Teo CG. The virology and serology of hepatitis: an overview. Communic Dis Rep 1992; 2: R109–R114. *Review. For reviews of epidemiology, control, diagnosis and management of viral hepatitis see pp R114–R120.*

Antibiotic-resistant pneumococci

Friedland IR, Klugman KP. Antibiotic-resistant pneumococcal disease in South African children. Am J Dis Child 1992; 146: 920–923. *The resistance of pneumococcus to beta-lactam antibiotics has increased alarmingly in South Africa. 40% of community-acquired isolates and 95% of hospital-acquired isolates were resistant to penicillin. For editorial see pp 912–916, and for report of increased prevalence in UK see Communic Dis Rep 1992; 2: R27–R43. For review of management of antibiotic-resistant pneumococci, see Pediatr Infect Dis J 1992; 11: 433–445.*

Tan TQ, Mason EO, Kaplan SL. Systemic infections due to *Streptococcus pneumoniae* relatively resistant to penicillin in a children's hospital: clinical management and outcome. Pediatrics 1992; 90: 928–933. *Documents 19 cases of serious infection with penicillin-resistant pneumococcus. For failure of chloramphenicol therapy in meningitis due to resistant pneumococci see Lancet 1992; 339: 405–408.*

Gastroenteritis

Cowden J. *Campylobacter:* epidemiological paradoxes. The vehicles for most cases of infection remain unknown. Br Med J 1992; 305: 132–133. *Editorial.*

Elliott EJ. Viral diarrhoeas in childhood. Electron microscopy has improved our understanding. Br Med J 1992; 305: 1111–1112. *Editorial. For enteric adenovirus infection see J Pediatr 1992; 120: 516–521.*

Human herpesvirus-6

Leach CT, Sumaya CV, Brown NA. Human herpesvirus-6: clinical implications of recently discovered, ubiquitous agent. J Pediatr 1992; 121: 173–181. *Review. For report of fatal case, see 120: 921–923.*

Linnavuori K, Peltola H, Hovi T. Serology versus clinical signs or symptoms and main laboratory findings in the diagnosis of exanthema subitum (roseola infantum). Pediatrics 1992; 89: 103–106. *Serological evidence of recent human herpesvirus-6 infection was obtained in 23 out of 25 (92%) cases.*

Pruksananonda P, Hall CB, Insel RA et al. Primary human herpesvirus 6 infection in young children. N Engl J Med 1992; 326: 1445–1450. *Primary infection with human herspesvirus-6 is the cause of acute febrile illness in young children. Such infection is associated with varied clinical manifestations, viraemia and the frequent persistence of the viral genome in mononuclear cells. For correspondence, see 327: 1099–1100.*

Intrauterine infection

Boppana SB, Pass RF, Britt WJ. Symptomatic congenital cytomegalovirus infection: neonatal morbidity and mortality. Pediatr Infect Dis J 1992; 11: 93–99. *Report of data in 106 neonates with symptomatic congenital cytomegalovirus (CMV) infection. For prenatal diagnosis of congenital CMV by virus isolation after amniocentesis, see pp 605–609.*

Fowler KB, Stagno S, Pass RF et al. The outcome of congenital cytomegalovirus infection in relation to maternal antibody status. N Engl J Med 1992; 326: 663–667. *The presence of maternal antibody to CMV before conception provides substantial protection against damaging congenital CMV infection in the newborn. For editorial, see pp 702–703.*

Hall SM. Congenital toxoplasmosis. Br Med J 1992; 305: 291–297. *Review. For cat ownership and toxoplasmosis, see Pediatrics 1992; 89; 1169–1172.*

McIntosh D, Isaacs D. Herpes simplex virus infection in pregnancy. Arch Dis Child 1992; 67: 1137–1138. *Review.*

Williamson WD, Demmler CJ, Percy AK et al. Progressive hearing loss in infants with asymptomatic congenital cytomegalovirus infection. Pediatrics 1992; 90: 862–866. *The audiologic outcome of 59 infants with asymptomatic congenital CMV infection was compared with 26 control infants. 8 of the 59 infected infants, but none of the controls, had congenital sensorineural hearing loss and longitudinal assessment showed that 5 of these 8 had further deterioration of their hearing loss.*

Meningitis

Feigin RD, McCracken GH, Klein JO. Diagnosis and management of meningitis. Pediatr Infect Dis J 1992; 11: 785–814. *Review. For the effect of duration on symptoms on outcome, see pp 694–701, and for review of pathogenesis and pathophysiology, see N Engl J Med 1992; 327: 864–872.*

Friedland IR, Paris MM, Rinderknecht S et al. Cranial computed tomographic scans have little impact on management of bacterial meningitis. Am J Dis Child 1992; 146: 1484–1487. *Computed tomography seldom reveals findings that require specific intervention.*

Mellor DH. The place of computed tomography and lumbar puncture in suspected bacterial meningitis. Arch Dis Child 1992; 67: 1417–1419. *Review.*

METABOLIC

Dixon MA, Leonard JV. Intercurrent illness in inborn errors of intermediary metabolism. Arch Dis Child 1992; 67: 1387–1391. *Review.*

Editorial. Excess water administration and hyponatraemic convulsions in infancy. Lancet 1992; 339: 153–155. *Review. See also* Br Med J *1992; 304: 1218–1222.*

Green A, Hall SM. Investigation of metabolic disorders resembling Reye's syndrome. Arch Dis Child 1992; 67: 1313–1317. *Review.*

Hale DE, Bennett MJ. Fatty acid oxidation disorders: a new class of metabolic diseases. J Pediatr 1992; 121: 1–11. *Review.*

Percy AK. Childhood metabolic disease with central nervous system involvement. Curr Opin Pediatr 1992; 4: 940–948. *Review.*

Sharples PM, Seckl JR, Human D et al. Plasma and cerebrospinal fluid arginine vasopressin in patients with and without fever. Arch Dis Child 1992; 67: 998–1002. *74% of febrile infected children were hyponatraemic (sodium <135 mmol/l) compared with only 8% of afebrile controls. Careful attention should be paid to fluid and electrolyte balance in all children with acute infections.*

Shoemaker JD, Lynch RE, Hoffmann JW et al. Misidentification of propionic acid as ethylene glycol in a patient with methylmalonic acidemia. J Pediatr 1992; 120: 417–421. *Severe metabolic acidosis caused suspicion of ethylene glycol poisoning. Re-examination of the serum showed that the chromatographic peak identified as ethylene glycol was actually due to propionic acid. Proof of a metabolic basis for the child's symptoms exonerated his mother of the charge of murder. See also pp 421–424.*

Walravens PA, Chakar A, Mokni R et al. Zinc supplements in breastfed infants. Lancet 1992; 340: 683–885. *The results of a zinc supplementation trial suggesting that among infants who were breast-fed for longer than 4 months, decreases in growth velocity may result partly from inadequate zinc intake. For correspondence, see pp 1416–1417.*

Wraith JE. Diagnosis and management of inborn errors of metabolism — an update. Arch Dis Child 1992; 67: 1231–1232. *Review.*

MISCELLANEOUS

Communication

Isaacman DJ, Purvis K, Gyuro J et al. Standardized instructions: do they improve communication of discharge information from the emergency department? Pediatrics 1992; 89: 1204–1208. *The addition of written instructions to standardized verbal instructions did not improve parental recall of discharge information.*

Rylance G. Should audio recordings of outpatient consultations be presented to patients? Arch Dis Child 1992; 67: 622–624. *Recording outpatient consultations helped parents and grandparents.*

Fever

Kluger MJ. Fever revisited. Pediatrics 1992; 90: 846–850. *Review. For fever phobia see Pediatrics 1992; 90: 851–854 and for data showing the need for rectal temperature measurement in infants see Arch Dis Child 1992; 67: 122–125.*

Intravenous fluid replacement

Huskisson L. Intravenous volume replacement: which fluid and why? Arch Dis Child 1992; 67: 649–653. *Review.*

Parotitis

Cohen HA, Gross S, Nussinovitch M et al. Recurrent parotitis. Arch Dis Child 1992; 67: 1036–1037. *Report of 11 children who had from 3 to 12 recurrences per year.*

NEONATOLOGY

Burman LG, Christensen P, Christensen K et al. Prevention of excess neonatal morbidity associated with group B streptococci by vaginal chlorhexidine disinfection during labour. Lancet 1992; 340: 65–69. *Chlorhexidine disinfection of the vagina during labour prevents neonatal disease. For prevention of group B streptococcal infection, see also Pediatr Infect Dis J 1992; 11: 179–183 and Pediatrics 1992; 90: 775–778.*

Chasnoff IJ. Cocaine, pregnancy, and the growing child. Curr Probl Pediatr 1992; 22: 302–321. *Review. See also N Engl J Med 1992; 327: 399–407.*

Gault DT. Vascular compromise in newborn infants. Arch Dis Child 1992; 67: 463–467. *Review.*

Greenough A, Milner AD. Respiratory support using patient triggered ventilation in the neonatal period. Arch Dis Child 1992; 67: 69–71. *Review.*

Lagercrantz H. What does the preterm infant breathe for? Controversies on apnoea of prematurity. Acta Paediatr 1992; 81: 733–736. *Review.*

Levene MI, Quinn MW. Use of sedatives and muscle relaxants in newborn babies receiving mechanical ventilation. Arch Dis Child 1992; 870–873. *Review.*

Marlow N. Do we need an Apgar score? Arch Dis Child 1992; 67: 765–769. *Review.*

Peled N, Dagan O, Babyn P et al. Gastric-outlet obstruction induced by prostaglandin therapy in neonates. N Engl J Med 1992; 327: 505–510. *The administration of prostaglandin E_1 to neonates can cause gastric-outlet obstruction due to antral hyperplasia.*

Sanchez L, Calvo M, Brock JH. Biological role of lactoferrin. Arch Dis Child 1992; 67: 657–661. *Review.*

Van Maldergem L, Jauniaux E, Fourneau C et al. Genetic causes of hydrops fetalis. Pediatrics 1992; 89: 81–86. *Genetic causes accounted for 35% of cases.*

Walter JH. Metabolic acidosis in newborn infants. Arch Dis Child 1992; 67: 767–769. *Review.*

Whitelaw A, Rivers RPA, Creighton L et al. Low dose intraventricular fibrinolytic treatment to prevent posthaemorrhagic hydrocephalus. Arch Dis Child 1992; 67: 12–14. *9 preterm infants with progressive ventricular dilation were treated with intraventricular infusion of streptokinase for 12–72 hours. All the infants survived and surgical shunting was required in only 1 (compared to expected figure of 5 or 6).*

Bronchopulmonary dysplasia

Ballard RA, Ballard PL, Creasy RK et al. Respiratory disease in very-low-birthweight infants after prenatal thyrotropin-releasing hormone and glucocorticoid. Lancet 1992; 339: 510–515. *Prenatal thyrotrophin-releasing hormone reduces the incidence of chronic lung disease amongst betamethasone-treated infants. For beneficial effect of fluid restriction, see* Eur J Pediatr 1992; 151: 295–299.

O'Neil EA, Chwals WJ, O'Shea MD. Dexamethasone treatment during ventilator dependency: possible life threatening gastrointestinal complications. Arch Dis Child 1992; 67: 10–11. *Report of 3 cases. For a report of adverse metabolic effects of dexamethasone, see pp 5–9.*

Jaundice

Rubo J, Albrecht K, Lasch P et al. High-dose intravenous immune globulin therapy for hyperbilirubinemia caused by Rh hemolytic disease. J Pediatr 1992; 121: 93–97. *This treatment, by a yet unknown mechanism, reduces serum bilirubin levels and the need for exchange transfusion.*

Watchko JF, Oski FA. Kernicterus in preterm newborns: past, present and future. Pediatrics 1992; 90: 707–715. *Review. For editorial, see pp 757–759.*

Respiratory distress syndrome (RDS)

Hallman M, Bry K, Hoppu K et al. Inositol supplementation in premature infants with respiratory distress syndrome. N Engl J Med 1992; 326: 1233–1239. *Inositol is a 6-carbon sugar alcohol which is a component of membrane phospholipids, and which influences organ maturation and cell function. Inositol supplementation in infants with RDS who are receiving parenteral nutrition during the first week of life was associated with increased survival without bronchopulmonary dysplasia and with a decreased incidence of retinopathy of prematurity. For editorial, see pp 1285–1287.*

Speer CP, Robertson B, Curstedt T et al. Randomized European multicenter trial of surfactant replacement therapy of severe neonatal respiratory distress syndrome: single versus multiple doses of Curosurf. Pediatrics 1992; 89: 13–20. *Treatment with multiple doses of surfactant is more effective than single-dose treatment in severe neonatal RDS. For symposium on synthetic surfactant (8 papers), see J Pediatr 1992; 120 (2 Part 2): S1–S50.*

The OSIRIS Collaborative Group. Early versus delayed neonatal administration of a synthetic surfactant — the judgment of OSIRIS. Lancet 1992; 340: 1363–1369. *The results suggest that early administration of exogenous surfactant to infants at high risk of RDS prevents both death and chronic lung disease, and reduces the risk of clinically important air leaks. See editorial on p 1387, and correspondence in 1993; 341: 172–174.*

NEPHROLOGY

Deal JE, Snell MF, Barratt TM et al. Renovascular disease in childhood. J Pediatr 1992; 121: 378–384. *Review of 54 cases referred for investigation of hypertension and who were found to have renovascular disease. In 8 cases it was associated with neurofibromatosis, in 3 with idiopathic hypercalcaemia and in 5 it followed an arteritic illness.*

Goldstein AR, White RHR, Akuse R. Long-term follow-up of childhood Henoch–Schönlein nephritis. Lancet 1992; 339: 280–282. *44% of patients who had nephritis, nephrotic or nephritic/nephrotic syndromes at onset have hypertension or impaired renal function. For pulmonary haemorrhage in Henoch–Schönlein purpura, see Pediatrics 1992; 89: 1177–1181.*

Perrone HC, dos Santos DR, Santos MV et al. Urolithiasis in childhood: metabolic evaluation. Pediatr Nephrol 1992; 6: 54–56. *There is an underlying metabolic abnormality in most cases.*

Haemolytic uraemic syndrome

Bergstein JM, Riley M, Bang NU. Role of plasminogen-activator inhibitor type 1 in the pathogenesis and outcome of the hemolytic uremic syndrome. N Engl J Med 1992; 327: 755–759. *Suggests, but does not prove that plasminogen-activator inhibitor type 1 is the circulating inhibitor of fibrinolysis in the haemolytic uraemic syndrome.*

Lopez EL, Devoto S, Fayad A et al. Association between severity of gastrointestinal prodrome and long-term prognosis in classic hemolytic-uremic syndrome. J Pediatr 1992; 120: 210–215. *The severity of the gastrointestinal prodrome reflects the severity of the extraintestinal acute microangiopathic process and the resulting long-term outcome.*

Urinary tract infection

Jakobsson B, Soderlundh S, Berg U. Diagnostic significance of ^{99m}Tc-dimercaptosuccinic acid (DMSA) scintigraphy in urinary tract infection. Arch Dis Child 1992; 67: 1338–1342. *A normal DMSA scan during or approximately 2 months after urinary tract infection indicates a low risk of finding significant pathology of the urinary tract.*

Rickwood AMK, Carty HM, McKendrick T et al. Current imaging of childhood urinary infections: prospective survey. Br Med J 1992; 304: 663–665. *Ultrasonography alone is inadequate for routine screening of childhood urinary infection. Further investigations remain advisable in infants, although in children they can be restricted to a minority who have positive ultrasound examinations or have had fever or vomiting. Radioisotope examinations largely eliminate the need for intravenous urography.*

Smith GC, Taylor CM. Recovery of protein from urine specimens collected in cotton wool. Arch Dis Child 1992; 67: 1486–1487. *Concentrations of albumin and retinol-binding protein decreased by 40 and 80% respectively within 15 minutes of contact with cotton wool, and cotton wool balls should not be used when investigating proteinuria.*

Vesicoureteric reflux (VUR)

Editorial. Vesicoureteric reflux and nephropathy. Lancet 1992; 339: 398–399. *Review.*

Kenda RB, Fettich JJ. Vesicoureteric reflux and renal scars in asymptomatic siblings of children with reflux. Arch Dis Child 1992; 67: 506–508. *The predictive value of positive family history alone in identifying VUR was 45%, and 23% of siblings with VUR were found to have renal scars.*

Steele BT, De Maria J. A new perspective on the natural history of vesicoureteric reflux. Pediatrics 1992; 90: 30–32. *VUR in children may be both a congenital abnormality, more common in boys, and an acquired abnormality, more common in girls.*

NEUROLOGY

Allsopp MR, Zaiwalla Z. Narcolepsy. Arch Dis Child 1992; 67: 302–306. *Report of 3 cases and review of management.*

Armstrong RW. Intrathecal baclofen and spasticity: what do we know and what do we need to know? Dev Med Child Neurol 1992; 34: 739–745. *Review.*

Bodensteiner JB, Hille MR, Riggs JE. Clinical features of vascular thrombosis following varicella. Am J Dis Child 1992; 146: 100–102. *Report of hemiparesis occurring 3–8 weeks after a primary infection in 5 children. See also Lancet 1992; 339: 1449–1450.*

Bushby KMD. Recent advances in understanding muscular dystrophy. Arch Dis Child 1992; 67: 1310–1312. *Review.*

Clayton-Smith J. Angelman's syndrome. Arch Dis Child 1992; 67: 889–891. *Review.*

Daoust-Roy J, Seshia SS. Benign neonatal sleep myoclonus. A differential diagnosis of neonatal seizures. Am J Dis Child 1992; 146: 1236–1241. *The features are myoclonic jerks only during sleep, abrupt and consistent cessation with arousal, absence of concomitant EEG changes and a good outcome. This disorder should be included in the differential diagnosis of neonatal seizures.*

Johnson SLJ, Hall DMB. Post-traumatic tremor in head injured children. Arch Dis Child 1992; 67: 227–228. *In 289 severely head-injured children, the prevalence of significant tremor was at least 45%. The tremor appeared within the first 18 months after injury, and in half the cases it subsequently subsided.*

Ropper AH. The Guillain–Barré syndrome. N Engl J Med 1992; 326: 1130–1136. *Review. For study showing that intravenous immune globulin is at least as effective as plasma exchange, see pp 1123–1129.*

Rothner AD. Classification, pathogenesis, evaluation, and management of headaches in children with adolescents. Curr Opin Pediatr 1992; 4:

949–956. *Review. For epidemiology of headache and migraine, see* Dev Med Child Neurol *1992; 34: 1095–1101.*

Stores G. Sleep problems. Arch Dis Child 1992; 67: 1420–1421. *Review.*

Cerebral palsy

Nicholson A, Alberman E. Cerebral palsy — an increasing contributor to severe mental retardation? Arch Dis Child 1992; 67: 1050–1055. *Review.*

Epilepsy

Berg AT, Shinnar S, Hauser A et al. A prospective study of recurrent febrile seizures. N Engl J Med 1992; 327: 1122–1127. *A shorter duration of fever before the initial febrile seizure and a lower temperature are associated with an increased risk of recurrence in children who have febrile seizures. For editorial, see pp 1161–1163, and for population-based birth cohort study of epilepsy in children under 10 in the UK, see* Br Med J *1992; 305: 857–861.*

Editorial. Diagnosing juvenile myoclonic epilepsy. Lancet 1992; 340: 759–760. *Review.*

Noetzel MJ, Blake JN. Seizures in children with congenital hydrocephalus: long-term outcome. Neurology 1992; 42: 1277–1281. *Indicates that medication can be safely discontinued in children with congenital hydrocephalus who are of normal intelligence and have been seizure-free on anticonvulsants for 3 years.*

Scher MS. Pediatric epilepsy. Curr Opin Pediatr 1992; 4: 921–929. *Review.*

Shinnar S, Maytal J, Krasnoff L et al. Recurrent status epilepticus in children. Ann Neurol 1992; 31: 598–604. *Prospective study of 95 cases; recurrent status epilepticus occurs mainly in children with an underlying neurological abnormality.*

OPHTHALMOLOGY

Casteels I, Harris CM, Shawkat F et al. Nystagmus in infancy. Br J Ophthalmol 1992; 76: 434–437. *Review.*

Retinopathy of prematurity

Batton DG, Roberts C, Trese M et al. Severe retinopathy of prematurity and steroid exposure. Pediatrics 1992; 90: 534–536. *More infants treated with dexamethasone for chronic lung disease needed cryotherapy for retinopathy. (In contrast, in another study, steroid therapy did not affect the number of infants who needed cryotherapy — see pp 529–533, and for editorial, see pp 646–647.)*

Clark DI, O'Brien C, Weindling AM et al. Initial experience of screening for retinopathy of prematurity. Arch Dis Child 1992; 67: 1233–1236. *Review. See also pp 860–867.*

Flynn JT, Bancalari E, Snyder ES et al. A cohort study of transcutaneous oxygen tension and the incidence and severity of retinopathy of prematurity. N Engl J Med 1992; 326: 1050–1054. *Supports an association between the incidence in severity of retinopathy of prematurity and the duration of exposure to arterial oxygen levels of 80 mmHg or higher. See editorial pp 1078–1080, and also Lancet 1992; 339: 961–962.*

Jacobson RM, Feinstein AR. Oxygen as a cause of blindness in premature infants: "autopsy" of a decade of errors in clinical epidemiologic research. J Clin Epidemiol 1992; 45: 1265–1287. *Review.*

Phelps DL. Retinopathy of prematurity. Curr Probl Pediatr 1992; 22: 349–371. *Reviews. For study of where the lesions are located in the retina, see Pediatrics 1992; 89: 648–653.*

ORTHOPAEDICS

Clarke NMP. Diagnosing congenital dislocation of the hip. A large trial of ultrasonography might help. Br Med J 1992; 304: 435–436. *Review. See correspondence pp 885–886 and see also Acta Paediatr 1992; 81: 177–181.*

Gardiner HM, Duncan AW. Radiological assessment of the effects of splinting on early hip development: results from a randomised controlled trial of abduction splinting vs sonographic surveillance. Pediatr Radiol 1992; 22: 159–162. *Hips that were splinted showed poorer epiphyseal maturation and iliac indentation compared with non-splinted hips by 6 months. Whether these differences have any long-term significance requires further study.*

Nishi Y, Hamamoto K, Kajiyama M et al. Effect of long term calcitonin therapy by injection and nasal spray on the incidence of fractures in osteogenesis imperfecta. J Pediatr 1992; 1221: 477–480. *In contrast to parenteral calcitonin, intranasal administration twice a week for 2 weeks, followed by 2 weeks of no therapy, is associated with improved compliance, and a reduced incidence of bone fractures.*

PSYCHIATRY

Creer TL, Stein REK, Rappaport L et al. Behavioral consequences of illness: childhood asthma as a model. Pediatrics 1992; 90: 808–815. *Review.*

Dare C. Change the family, change the child? Arch Dis Child 1992; 67: 643–648. *Review of family therapy.*

Gillberg CL. Autism and autistic-like conditions: subclasses among disorders of empathy. J Child Psychol Psychiatry 1992; 33: 813–842. *Review.*

Green J. Inpatient psychiatry units. Arch Dis Child 1992; 67: 1120–1123. *Review.*

Canning EH, Hanser SB, Shade KA et al. Mental disorders in chronically ill children: parent–child discrepancy and physician identification. Pediatrics 1992; 90: 692–696. *In 83 children with chronic diseases, the incidence of psychiatric disorders depended upon whether information had been obtained from the child, the parent or the doctor. Doctors' ratings agreed significantly with children's reports but not with parental reports, suggesting that doctors are sensitive to children's concerns but may underestimate the value and importance of parents' reports.*

Lask B. Psychological treatments for childhood asthma. Arch Dis Child 1992; 67: 891. *Review.*

Meadow R. Difficult and unlikeable parents. Arch Dis Child 1992; 67: 697–702. *Doctors of all grades understood why parents behaved in awkward ways, but lacked strategies for dealing with them.*

Prendergast M. Types of psychiatric treatment. Drug treatment. Arch Dis Child 1992; 67: 1488–1494. *Review.*

Rantakallio P, Koiranen M, Mottonen J. Association of perinatal events, epilepsy, and central nervous system trauma with juvenile delinquency. Arch Dis Child 1992; 67: 1459–1461. *Previous central nervous system (CNS) trauma may be a cause of delinquency. Alternatively, the type of behaviour pursued by males who are likely to commit a violent crime will expose them more often to accidents which can result in CNS trauma.*

Sturge C. Dealing with the courts and parenting breakdown. Arch Dis Child 1992; 67: 745–750. *Review.*

Swadi H. Drug abuse in children and adolescents: an update. Arch Dis Child 1992; 67: 1245–1246. *Review.*

Szatmari P. Asperger's syndrome. Curr Opin Pediatr 1992; 4: 616–622. *Review.*

Trowell J. Types of psychiatric treatment. Individual psychotherapy. Arch Dis Child 1992; 67: 336–339. *Review.*

Vereker MI. Chronic fatigue syndrome: a joint paediatric–psychiatric approach. Arch Dis Child 1992; 67: 550–555. *Review.*

RADIOLOGY

Carty H. Pediatric musculoskeletal radiology. Curr Opin Pediatr 1992; 4: 21–29. *Review.*

Chapman S. The radiological dating of injuries. Arch Dis Child 1992; 67: 1063–1065. *Review.*

RESPIRATORY

De Blic J, Scheinmann P. Fibreoptic bronchoscopy in infants. Arch Dis Child 1992; 67: 159–161. *Review.*

Editorial. Indoor air pollution and acute respiratory infections in children. Lancet 1992; 339: 396–398. *Review.*

Editorial. Reversibility of airflow obstruction: FEV_1 vs peak flow. Lancet 1992; 340: 85–86. *Review.*

Editorial. Indoor air pollution and acute respiratory infections in children. Lancet 1992; 339: 396–398. *Review.*

Loughlin GM. Obstructive sleep apnea in children. Adv Pediatr 1992; 39: 307–336.

Murray M, Webb MSC, O'Callaghan C et al. Respiratory status and allergy after bronchiolitis. Arch Dis Child 1992; 67: 482–487. *73 children admitted to hospital with acute bronchiolitis were reviewed 5 years later and compared with a matched control group. In the post-bronchiolitis group there was a highly significant increase in respiratory symptoms including wheezing (42.5 versus 15%).*

Schuh S, Johnson D, Canny G et al. Efficacy of adding nebulized ipratropium bromide to nebulized albuterol therapy in acute bronchiolitis. Pediatrics 1992; 90: 920–923. *The addition of nebulized ipratropium offers no further clinical benefit compared with salbutamol alone in moderately severe bronchiolitis. See also Arch Dis Child 1992; 67: 289–293. For review of the respiratory syncytial virus and bronchiolitis see Eur J Pediatr 1992; 141: 638–651.*

Weese-Mayer DE, Silvestri JM, Menzies LJ et al. Congenital central hypoventilation syndrome: diagnosis, management, and long-term outcome in thirty-two children. J Pediatr; 120: 381–387. *Review.*

Asthma

Bentur L, Canny GJ, Shields MD. Controlled trial of nebulized albuterol in children younger than 2 years of age with acute asthma. Pediatrics

1992; 89: 133–137. *After 2 nebulizations, the salbutamol-treated patients had a greater improvement in clinical status than the placebo group.*

Coutts JAP, Gibson NA, Paton JY. Measuring compliance with inhaled medication in asthma. Arch Dis Child 1992; 67: 332–333. *An electronic inhaler timer device, which electronically counts and times each actuation, documented underuse of treatment in 55% of study days and overuse in only 2%.*

Keeley D. Large volume plastic spacers in asthma. Should be used more. Br Med J 1992; 304: 598–599. *Editorial. See also* Arch Dis Child *1992; 67: 580–585, and for drug delivery by jet nebulizer see* Arch Dis Child *1992; 67: 586–591.*

Lloyd BW, Ali MH. How useful do parents find home peak flow monitoring for children with asthma? Br Med J 1992; 305: 1128–1129. *The authors defined a 'danger' peak flow level as about 60% of the child's best, and parents found this a useful figure to help them judge their child's response to bronchodilators.*

MacDonald JB. Nocturnal asthma. What happens to the airways at night? Br Med J 1992; 304: 998–999. *Review.*

McFadden ER, Gilbert IA. Asthma. N Engl J Med 1992; 327: 1928–1937. *Review.*

Noble V, Ruggins NR, Everard ML et al. Inhaled budesonide for chronic wheezing under 18 months of age. Arch Dis Child 1992; 67: 285–288. *Budesonide given through a large-volume spacer (Nebuhaler) with an attached Laerdal facemask was an effective treatment for infants who needed prophylaxis for wheezing.*

Pattemore PK, Johnston SL, Bardin PG. Viruses as precipitants of asthma symptoms. I. Epidemiology. Clin Exp Allergy 1992; 22: 325–336. *Review.*

Springer C, Avital A, Noviski N et al. Role of infection in the middle lobe syndrome in asthma. Arch Dis Child 1992; 67: 592–594. *Long-standing right middle lobe collapse in asthmatic children is often associated with bacterial infection.*

Warner J.O. Asthma: a follow up statement from an international paediatric asthma consensus group. Arch Dis Child 1992; 67: 240–248. *Consensus statement.*

Wilson NM, Phagoo SB, Silverman M. Atopy, bronchial responsiveness, and symptoms in wheezy 3 year olds. Arch Dis Child 1992; 67: 491–495. *In this hospital-based study, acute wheeze associated with colds in the first 3 years of life was independent of the finding of atopy, and bronchial responsiveness in this age group may have a different pathogenesis from that in older subjects.*

Cystic fibrosis

Hubbard RC, McElvaney NG, Birrer P et al. A preliminary study of aerosolized recombinant human deoxyribonuclease I in the treatment of cystic fibrosis. N Engl J Med 1992; 326: 812–815. *Treatment was associated with significant improvement of lung function, was easily administered, and well-tolerated.*

Stanghelle JK, Skyberg D, Haanaes OC. Eight-year follow-up of pulmonary function and oxygen uptake during exercise in 16-year-old males with cystic fibrosis. Acta Paediatr 1992; 81: 527–531. *Regular physical exercise has a beneficial long-term effect.*

Tizzano EF, Buchwald M. Cystic fibrosis: beyond the gene to therapy. J Pediatr 1992; 120: 337–349. *Review.*

Croup

Tibballs J, Shann FA, Landau LI. Placebo-controlled trial of prednisolone in children intubated for croup. Lancet 1992; 340: 745–748. *Prednisolone 1 mg/kg 12-hourly by nasogastric tube until 24 hours after extubation reduced the duration of intubation and the need for reintubation in children intubated for croup.*

RHEUMATOLOGY

Giannini EH, Brewer EJ, Kuzmina N et al. Methotrexate in resistant juvenile rheumatoid arthritis. N Engl J Med 1992; 326: 1043–1049. *Methotrexate given weekly in low doses is an effective treatment for children with resistant juvenile rheumatoid arthritis, and at least in the short term this regimen is safe. For editorial, see pp 1077–1078.*

Schaller JG. Rheumatic diseases of children. Curr Opin Pediatr 1992; 4: 1017–1024. *Review.*

Schneider R, Lang BA, Reilly BJ et al. Prognostic indicators of joint destruction in systemic-onset juvenile rheumatoid arthritis. J Pediatr 1992; 120: 200–205. *Patients at high risk for the development of destructive arthritis may be identified within 6 months of disease onset, thereby indicating the need for more aggressive early therapy.*

Walco GA, Varni JW, Ilowite NT. Cognitive-behavioural pain management in children with juvenile rheumatoid arthritis. Pediatrics 1992; 89: 1075–1079. *Cognitive-behavioural interventions (progressive muscle relaxation, meditative breathing exercises and guided imagery) for pain are an effective adjunct to standard pharmacological treatment.*

SURGERY

Atwell JD, Spargo PM. The provision of safe surgery for children. Arch Dis Child 1992; 67: 345–349. *Review.*

Bhisitkul DM, Listernick R, Shkolnik A et al. Clinical application of ultrasonography in the diagnosis of intussusception. J Pediatr 1992; 121: 182–186. *Children at low risk of having intussusception on the basis of clinical symptoms should initially have an ultrasound examination; patients at high risk should have an immediate barium enema.*

Devane SP, Coombes R, Smith VV et al. Persistent gastrointestinal symptoms after correction of malrotation. Arch Dis Child 1992; 67: 218–221. *Persistence of symptoms after surgical correction of a malrotation is associated with a motility disturbance which seems to be due to a defect of intrinsic enteric innervation.*

Fine RN. Diagnosis and treatment of fetal urinary tract abnormalities. J Pediatr 1992; 121: 333–341. *Review.*

Sethia B. Current status of definitive surgery for congenital heart disease. Arch Dis Child 1992; 67: 981–984. *Annotation. Review.*

Stringer MD, Pledger G, Drake DP. Childhood deaths from intussusception in England and Wales, 1984–9. Br Med J 1992; 304: 737–739. *Study of 33 deaths, median age 7 months. Avoidable factors were excessive delay in diagnosis, inadequate intravenous fluid and antibiotic therapy, delay in recognizing recurrent or residual intussusception after hydrostatic reduction and surgical complications.*

Transplantation

Chiyende J, Mowat AP. Liver transplantation. Arch Dis Child 1992; 67: 1124–1127. *Review. See also* Br Med J *1992; 304: 416–421.*

Grimm PC, Ettenger R. Pediatric renal transplantation. Adv Pediatr 1992: 39: 441–493. *Review. See also* N Engl J Med *1992; 326: 1727–1732.*

Madden BP, Hodson ME, Tsang V et al. Intermediate-term results of heart-lung transplantation for cystic fibrosis. Lancet 1992; 339: 1583–1587. *The main obstacles to be overcome are the shortage of donor organs and the complication of obliterative bronchiolitis.*

THERAPEUTICS

Clogg DK. Varicella in children receiving steroids for asthma: risks and management. Pediatr Infect Dis J 1992; 11: 419–420. *Children who receive short-term steroid therapy for asthma are at increased risk of serious complications or death from varicella. Possible strategies are discussed.*

Editorial. Controversy about chickenpox. Lancet 1992; 340: 639–340. *Review of the value and cost of oral acyclovir in otherwise healthy children with chickenpox. See also J Pediatr 1992; 120: 627–633, and for complications of varicella which required hospitalization in previously healthy children, see Pediatr Infect Dis J 1992; 11: 441–445.*

Editorial. Pacifiers, passive behaviour, and pain. Lancet 1992; 339: 275–276. *Review.*

Ezekowitz RAB, Mulliken JB, Folkman J. Interferon Alfa-2a therapy for life-threatening hemangiomas of infancy. N Engl J Med 1992; 326: 1456–1463. *Treatment was associated with benefit. For editorial, see pp 1491–1493, and for correspondence, see 327: 1321–1322.*

Garland JS, Dunne M, Havens P et al. Peripheral intravenous catheter complications in critically ill children: a prospective study. Pediatrics 1992: 89: 1145–1150. *Replacing catheters in critically ill children every 72 hours would not decrease phlebitis, bacterial colonization, or catheter-induced sepsis. Catheters could be safely maintained for up to 144 hours in critically ill children.*

Golding J, Greenwood, R, Birmingham K et al. Childhood cancer, intramuscular vitamin K, and pethidine given during labour. Br Med J 1992; 305: 341–346. *This study reported a significant association between intramuscular vitamin K and the subsequent development of childhood cancer. There was no significantly increased risk for children who had been given oral vitamin K or whether mother had received pethidine in labour. See editorial on pp 326–327 and correspondence on pp 709–711.*

Igarashi M, May WN, Golden GS. Pharmacologic treatment of childhood migraine. J Pediatr 1992; 120: 653–657. *Review.*

Kinmonth A-L, Fulton Y, Campbell MJ. Management of feverish children at home. Br Med J 1992; 305: 1134–1136. *Advice to give paracetamol is more effective than sponging or unwrapping in controlling temperature in children at home and is more acceptable to parents.*

Lambert J, Mobassaleh M, Grand J et al. Efficacy of cimetidine for gastric acid suppression in pediatric patients. J Pediatr 1992; 120: 474–478. *Recommended doses of cimetidine for children may not be sufficient for adequate gastric acid suppression.*

Parke TJ, Stevens JE, Rice ASC et al. Metabolic acidosis and fatal myocardial failure after propofol infusion in children: five case reports. Br Med J 1992; 305: 613–616. *Report of 5 children who were intubated because of croup or bronchiolitis. Sedation with propofol was associated with the development of lipaemic serum, increasing metabolic acidosis, progressive myocardial failure and death in all 5. For correspondence, see pp 952–954.*

Stiehm ER. Recent progress in the use of intravenous immunoglobulin. Curr Probl Pediatr 1992; 22: 335–348. *Review. For use in neonatal sepsis, see* Adv Pediatr *1992; 39: 71–99 and* J Pediatr *1992; 121: 401–404 and 434–443.*

TROPICAL

Aaby P. Influence of cross-sex transmission on measles mortality in rural Senegal. Lancet 1992; 340: 388–391. *Measles infection contracted from a person of the opposite sex is more severe, although the reason for this is not understood. See also* Br Med J *1992; 304: 284–287.*

Berkowitz FE. Infections in children with severe protein-energy malnutrition. Pediatr Infect Dis J 1992; 11: 750–759. *Review.*

Forgie IM, Campbell H, Lloyd-Evans N. Etiology of acute lower respiratory tract infections in children in a rural community in the Gambia. Pediatr Infect Dis J 1992; 11: 466–473. *In the absence of an outbreak of respiratory syncytial virus the viral agents recovered most often were influenza A and adenoviruses.*

Gunston GD, Burkimsher D, Malan H et al. Reversible cerebral shrinkage in kwashiorkor: an MRI study. Arch Dis Child 1992; 67: 1030–1032. *Brain shrinkage was present on admission in all 12 children who were studied. The shrinkage reversed rapidly with nutritional rehabilitation. (For bone turnover in malnourished children, see* Lancet *1992; 340: 1493–1496.)*

Hayes EB, Gubler DJ. Dengue and dengue hemorrhagic fever. Pediatr Infect Dis J 1992; 11: 311–317. *Review.*

Jelliffe DB, Jelliffe EF. Causation of kwashiorkor: toward a multifactorial consensus. Pediatrics 1992; 90: 110–113. *Review.*

Lackritz EM Campbell CC, Ruebush Trenton K et al. Effect of blood transfusion on survival among children in a Kenyan hospital. Lancet 1992; 340: 524–528. *The frequency of blood transfusion can be reduced and survival enhanced by targeting blood to those children with severe anaemia and clinical signs of respiratory distress, and by using transfusion early in the course of hospitalization.*

Redd SC, Bloland PB, Kazembe PN et al. Usefulness of clinical case-definitions in guiding therapy for African children with malaria or pneumonia. Lancet 1992; 340: 1140–1143. *Children who satisfy the malaria and pneumonia clinical definitions need treatment for both disorders. For correspondence, see* Lancet *1993; 341: 304–305.*

Simoes EAF, McGrath EJ. Recognition of pneumonia by primary health care workers in Swaziland with a simple clinical algorithm. Lancet 1992;

340: 1502–1503. *Dangerous signs of stridor and abnormal sleepiness were poorly recognized by health care workers, but severe undernutrition, tachypnoea and chest wall indrawing were well-recognized. See also* Pediatr Infect Dis J *1992; 11: 77–81. For discussion of World Health Organization (WHO) definition of tachypnoea, see 339: 176–177.*

Snow RW, Armstrong JRM, Forster D et al. Childhood deaths in Africa: use and limitations of verbal autopsies. Lancet 1992; 340: 351–355. *The verbal autopsy (VA) is an epidemiological tool to ascribe causes of death by interviewing bereaved relatives of children who were not under medical supervision at the time of death. Common causes of death were detected by VA with specificities greater than 80%, but malaria, anaemia, acute respiratory tract infection, gastroenteritis and meningitis were detected with sensitivities of less than 50%.*

Gastroenteritis

Bhandari N, Bhan MK, Sazawal S. Mortality associated with acute watery diarrhea, dysentery and persistent diarrhea in rural North India. Acta Paediatr 1992; 381 (suppl): 3–6. *One of 28 papers in a supplement on persistent diarrhoea, with papers on epidemiology, sociobehavioural aspects, pathogenesis, management and effects on childhood mortality.*

Costello AM de L, Bhutta TI. Antidiarrhoeal drugs for acute diarrhoea in children. None work, and many may be dangerous. Br Med J 1992; 304: 1–2. *Review.*

Editorial. Cereal-based oral rehydration solutions — bridging the gap between fluid and food. Lancet 1992; 339: 219–220. *Review.*

Gore SM, Fontaine O, Pierce NF. Impact of rice based oral rehydration solution on stool output and duration of diarrhoea: meta-analysis of 13 clinical trials. Br Med J 1992; 304: 287–291. *The benefit of rice oral rehydration salts solution for patients with cholera is sufficiently great to warrant its use in such patients. The benefit is considerably smaller for children with acute, non-cholera diarrhoea and should be more precisely defined before its practical value can be judged.*

Immunization

Editorial. Typhoid vaccination: weighing the options. Lancet 1992; 340: 341–342. *Reviews.*

Vitamin A

Daulaire NMP, Starbuck ES, Houston RM et al. Childhood mortality after a high dose of vitamin A in a high risk population. Br Med J 1992; 304:

207–210. *The risk of death for children under 5 years in supplemented communities was 26% lower than in unsupplemented communities. For study reporting lack of effect on survival see* Lancet *1992; 340: 267–271, for report of a WHO/UNICEF conference, see* Lancet *1992; 339: 864, and for study of vitamin A supplementation in Ghana, see* Lancet *1992; 339: 361–362 and 1302–1303.*

Editorial. Detecting vitamin A deficiency early. Lancet 1992; 339: 1514–1516. *Review.*

Index

Italic page numbers refer to the literature review section